# SAS® Programming for R Users

## Jordan Bakerman

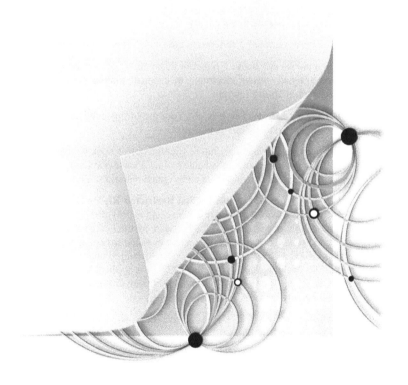

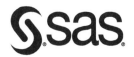 sas.com/books

The correct bibliographic citation for this manual is as follows: SAS Institute Inc. 2019. *SAS® Programming for R Users*. Cary, NC: SAS Institute Inc.

**SAS® Programming for R Users**

Copyright © 2019, SAS Institute Inc., Cary, NC, USA

ISBN 978-1-64295-715-0 (Paperback)
ISBN 978-1-64295-713-6 (PDF)

All Rights Reserved. Produced in the United States of America.

SAS Institute Inc., SAS Campus Drive, Cary, NC 27513-2414

December 2019

# Contents

# About This Book

## What Does This Book Cover?

SAS and R are both important tools for data analysis. SAS is a programming language as well as a suite of software solutions that can be used for data access, data management, data analytics, statistical analysis, and data presentation. SAS can handle large amounts of data and perform almost any data analysis task that is required by researchers and companies of any size. On the other hand, R is a free, open-source tool that is mostly used by the research community for statistical analysis, graphing, and reporting.

By some accounts, R is a more difficult programming language to learn than SAS. If you have learned how to perform analytical tasks in R and want to know how to perform the same tasks in SAS, then this is the book for you. This book covers a wide range of topics including the basics of the SAS programming language, how to import data, how to create new variables, random number generation, linear modeling, Interactive Matrix Language (IML), and many other SAS procedures. This book also covers how to write R code directly in the SAS code editor for seamless integration between the two tools.

This book is based on the free video course "SAS® Programming for R Users" offered by SAS Education and also available on Lynda.com. You may prefer to follow along with the videos, which offer more practice exercises and example scenarios than are contained in this book. At the end of each chapter, you will find questions and exercises to test your knowledge.

## Is This Book for You?

This book is designed for experienced R users who want to transfer their programming skills to SAS. Emphasis is on programming and not statistical theory or interpretation. You will learn how to write programs in SAS that replicate familiar functions and capabilities in R. You will also learn how to call R from SAS using IML.

## What Are the Prerequisites for This Book?

Readers should have knowledge of plotting, manipulating data, iterative processing, creating functions, applying functions, linear models, generalized linear models, mixed models, stepwise model selection, matrix algebra, and statistical simulations.

## What Should You Know about the Examples?

This book includes tutorials for you to follow to gain hands-on experience with SAS.

### Software Used to Develop the Book's Content

The software used to develop this book's content includes SAS 9.4 and SAS® Enterprise Miner™.

### Example Code and Data

You can access the example code and data for this book by linking to its author page at support.sas.com/bakerman.

## SAS University Edition

Many of the advanced techniques for working with R in this book are not compatible with SAS University Edition. If you are using SAS University Edition to access data and run your programs, then please check the SAS University Edition page to ensure that the software contains the product or products that you need to run the code: www.sas.com/universityedition.

## Where Are the Exercise Solutions?

The exercise solutions can be found immediately following the exercises in the same chapter.

## We Want to Hear from You

SAS Press books are written *by* SAS Users *for* SAS Users. We welcome your participation in their development and your feedback on SAS Press books that you are using. Please visit sas.com/books to do the following:

- Sign up to review a book
- Recommend a topic
- Request information on how to become a SAS Press author
- Provide feedback on a book

Do you have questions about a SAS Press book that you are reading? Contact the author through saspress@sas.com or https://support.sas.com/author_feedback.

SAS has many resources to help you find answers and expand your knowledge. If you need additional help, see our list of resources: sas.com/books.

Learn more about this author by visiting his author page at support.sas.com/bakerman. There you can download free book excerpts, access example code and data, read the latest reviews, get updates, and more.

# Chapter 1: Introduction to SAS

## Introduction

If you are reading this book, you most likely have never used SAS or have limited experience with SAS. So, what is SAS? SAS is a suite of business solutions and technologies to help organizations solve business problems. That is the official slogan, but it's much broader than that. SAS is for anyone who needs to manage data or create advanced analytics models. SAS is powered by high-performance analytics, which are thoroughly tested before coming to market. SAS enables you to access and manage data across multiple sources as well as perform analyses and deliver information across your organization.

The functionality of SAS is built around four data-driven tasks that are common to virtually any application:

- data access

- data management

- data analysis, including creating inferential models

- data presentation

In SAS, all of our data sets are going to be on disk, which means they are on the hard drive. This is a little bit different coming from R. Data sets in SAS will need to be read into memory as needed, which will be seamless behind-the-scenes.

## SAS Versus R

R is an object-oriented programming language. Results of a function are stored in an object and desired results are pulled from the object as needed. SAS revolves around the data table and uses procedures to create and print output. Results can be saved to a new data table.

In this section, we will briefly compare SAS and R in a general way to help you learn additional SAS programming skills independently. Look at Table 1.1, which outlines some of the major differences between SAS and R.

**Table 1.1: SAS Versus R**

| SAS | R |
| --- | --- |
| Script compiler | Command line interpreter |
| Primarily driven by the data table and procedures | Object-oriented |
| Not case-sensitive | Case-sensitive |

Here are a few other things about SAS to note:

- SAS has the flexibility to interact with objects. However, this book focuses on procedural methods.
- SAS does not have a command line. Code must be run in order to return results.

## SAS Programs

A *SAS program* is a sequence of one or more steps. A *step* is a sequence of SAS statements. There are only two types of steps in SAS: DATA and PROC steps.

- **DATA** steps read from an input source and create a SAS data set.
- **PROC** steps read and process a SAS data set, often generating an output report. Procedures can be called an umbrella term. They are what carry out the global analysis. Think of a PROC step as a function in R.

Every step has a beginning and ending boundary. SAS steps begin with either of the following statements:

- a DATA statement
- a PROC statement

After a DATA or PROC statement, there can be additional SAS statements that contain keywords that requests SAS to perform an operation or give information to the system. Think of them as additional arguments to a procedure. Statements always end with a semicolon!

SAS options are additional arguments and they are specific to SAS statements. Unfortunately, there is no rule to say what is a statement versus what is an option. Understanding the difference comes with a little bit of experience. Options can be used to do the following:

- generate additional output like results and plots
- save output to a SAS data table
- alter the analytical method

SAS detects the end of a step when it encounters one of the following statements:

- a RUN statement (for most steps)
- a QUIT statement (for some procedures)

Most SAS steps end with a RUN statement. Think of the RUN statement as the right parentheses of an R function. Table 1.2 shows an example of a SAS program that has a DATA step and a PROC step. You can see that both SAS statements end with RUN statements, while the R functions begin and end with parentheses.

Table 1.2: SAS Program Versus R Program

| SAS Program | R Program |
|---|---|
| ```
data work.newemps;
 infile "&path\newemps.csv" dlm=',';
 input First $ Last $ Title $ Salary;
run;

proc print data=work.newemps;
run;
``` | ```
work.newemps = read.csv
 ("C:/Users/username/
 Desktop/work.newemps.csv")
print(work.newemps)
``` |

## SAS Syntax Rules

SAS statements usually begin with a keyword, and always end with a semicolon. Keywords identify the type of statement, and semicolons end the statement.

A syntax error is an error in the spelling or grammar of a SAS statement. SAS finds syntax errors as it compiles each SAS statement, before execution begins. Common examples of syntax errors include:

- misspelled keywords
- unmatched quotation marks
- invalid options
- missing semicolons

The Enhanced Editor in some SAS interfaces uses the color red to indicate a potential error in your SAS code. Notice in Figure 1.1 that the misspelled word D-A-A-T is displayed in red. This misspelling affects other statements following it because those statements are only permitted in a DATA step, and this is not recognized as such.

Figure 1.1: SAS Code with Errors

```
daat work.newsalesemps;
   length First_Name $ 12
          Last_Name $ 18 Job_Title $ 25;
   infile "&path\newemps.csv" dlm=',';
   input First_Name $ Last_Name $
          Job_Title $ Salary;
run;

proc print data=work.newsalesemps
run;

proc means data=work.newsalesemps average min;
   var Salary;
run;
```

The RUN statement in the PROC PRINT step is not the correct font or color in Figure 1.1. Code can contain incorrect keywords for options. The word "average" in the PROC MEANS statement is also the wrong font and color, because "average" is not recognized by the PROC MEANS statement. (MEAN is the correct word.) Error messages are written to the SAS log to describe syntax errors.

> **Tip:** Bookmark the SAS Documentation page at support.sas.com/documentation. You can look up procedures, statements, options, analytical methods, and any type of SAS syntax.

## Comments

R comments do not have an end and simply comment out everything to the right of the # symbol. SAS comments are more functional. Program 1.1 contains four comments.

**Program 1.1: Comment Types**

```
|*---------------------------------------*|
|   This program creates and uses the    |   ❶
|   data set called work.newsalesemps.   |
|*---------------------------------------*;
data work.newsalesemps;
    length First_Name $ 12 Last_Name $ 18Job_Title $ 25;
    infile "&path\newemps.csv" dlm=',';
    input First_Name $ Last_Name $ Job_Title $ Salary /*numeric*/;   ❷
run;
   /*
proc print data=work.newsalesemps;   ❸
run;
   */
proc means data=work.newsalesemps;
    *var Salary;   ❹
run;
```

❶ The first comment describes the program.

❷ The second comment is within a statement.

❸ The third comment is commenting out a step.

❹ The fourth comment is commenting out a statement.

To comment multiple lines simultaneously in SAS, highlight the lines. Hold down the Ctrl key and press /. To uncomment, highlight the lines. Hold down the Ctrl and Shift keys and press /.

## SAS Interfaces

Since its inception over 40 years ago, SAS software has evolved significantly with changes in computer technology. This evolution resulted in three unique SAS interfaces:

1.  SAS windowing environment
2.  SAS Enterprise Guide
3.  SAS Studio

The SAS windowing environment is the original interface that is used to access, manage, analyze, and report data. For experienced programmers, the windowing environment might feel the most natural because it is the most basic interface of SAS. It provides an Editor window in which you can write and submit code without the use of any point-and-click features.

SAS Enterprise Guide is configured to access SAS on a local or remote server. SAS Enterprise Guide has point-and-click wizards and tasks for SAS procedures and a robust programming interface.

SAS Studio is the newest interface. It is a web-based interface to SAS that you can use on any computer. It combines functionality from both the windowing environment and Enterprise Guide. SAS Studio is consistent, available, and assistive. You learn one interface that you can use throughout your career, as a student, an individual SAS user or consultant, a departmental user, and an enterprise user. You can use the same interface wherever you need it (a Mac in a dorm, a Windows desktop at work, a laptop at home, and an iPad on the road). For programmers, the code is front and center, but you can use point-and-click functions such as code-generating tasks or process flows to help, if you need them.

No matter which SAS interface you use, the SAS programming is the same. In addition, they all offer these same basic programming tools:

- an Editor window where you write and submit SAS code
- a log where you view messages from SAS
- a page to view your results

However, in this book, we will focus on using SAS Studio because of its accessibility and features. SAS Studio can be accessed from any browser. After you access the interface from the browser, you can run a program and SAS Studio automatically connects to SAS on your machine. The analysis is run on the machine, and then the results are brought back to the browsers for you to see.

SAS University Edition is free SAS software that can be used for teaching and learning statistics and quantitative methods. It is designed for those who want easy access to statistical software. SAS University Edition uses the SAS Studio interface and gives you access to the following products:

- **Base SAS**: The foundation for all SAS software. It provides a highly flexible, highly extensible, fourth-generation programming language and a rich library of programming procedures.
- **SAS/ACCESS**: Seamlessly connect with your data no matter where it resides or how it is saved. SAS/ACCESS provides tools to easily access external data.
- **SAS/STAT**: Provides a wide variety of statistical methods and techniques.
- **SAS/IML**: A matrix programming language for more specialized analyses.
- **SAS/ETS**: A suite of time series forecasting procedures. SAS University Edition offers only the TIMEDATA, TIMESERIES, ARIMA, ESM, UCM, and TIMEID procedures.

**Note:** To run R with SAS, R must be installed on the same machine as SAS. Because SAS University Edition installs on a virtual machine where R cannot be installed, R cannot be used with SAS University Edition.

## SAS Studio Interface

Let's look at the SAS Studio interface. Open your SAS Studio session. It should look similar to Figure 1.2.

**Figure 1.2: SAS Studio Interface**

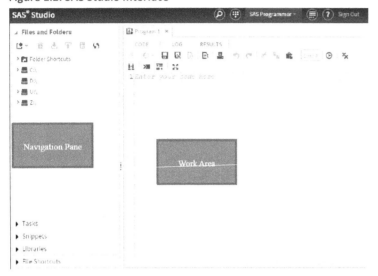

The SAS Studio interface is separated into the Navigation pane on the left and the Work area on the right, also called the Code Editor. The Work area displays your programs with tabs for Code, Log, and Results. The Navigation pane provides easy access to your folders and libraries that contain your permanent and temporary data sets. The Files and Folders tab is displayed by default. It automatically maps to the drives on your computer to give you quick access to load data sets and SAS programs.

Click the **Libraries** tab in the Navigation pane and select **My Libraries**, as shown in Figure 1.3.

**Figure 1.3: My Libraries**

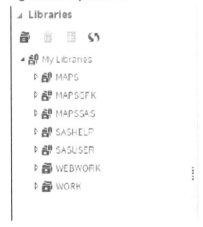

The Libraries are where you will store all of your data. Notice that they are separated by category. The libraries **MAPS** through **WEBWORK** are permanent libraries. The data displayed in each library is a permanent data set, which users can use at their convenience. Whatever data you save in these libraries will be saved after you close your SAS session. The **Work** library is a temporary library. Any data saved to the **Work** library by the user is deleted when the user closes the SAS session. In a later demonstration, you see how to save a new data set to the **Work** library and create a new permanent library. A new permanent library enables the user to load external data a single time and update or use the data table each new session. This heavily reduces the load time and cleaning time of your data because it is done only once.

Open the **Sashelp** library and navigate to the **cars** data set. Double-click the data set to open it in the Table Viewer in the Work area. The **cars** data set contains 428 total rows of data and 15 columns or variables. It is a sample of cars from the 1993 *Consumer Reports* magazine. You can use the arrows in the upper right to navigate between pages or the scroll bar at the bottom of the data table to change your view of the data. In the Columns area of the Table Viewer in Figure 1.4, notice that all columns are selected by default. Simply clear the check box from a column to remove the column from the viewer.

Figure 1.4: Cars Data Set

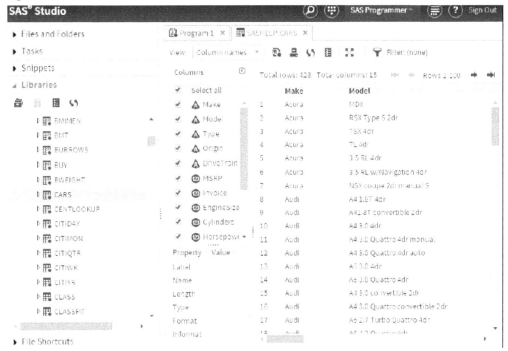

Clear the **Select all** check box and then select **Make**, **Model**, **Type**, **Origin**, **MSRP**, and **Invoice**.

To customize the view of the data table, select the arrow next to **Columns** to hide the columns area and then select the **Maximize View** icon. Your screen should now show only the selected columns, as shown in Figure 1.5.

Figure 1.5: Maximize View

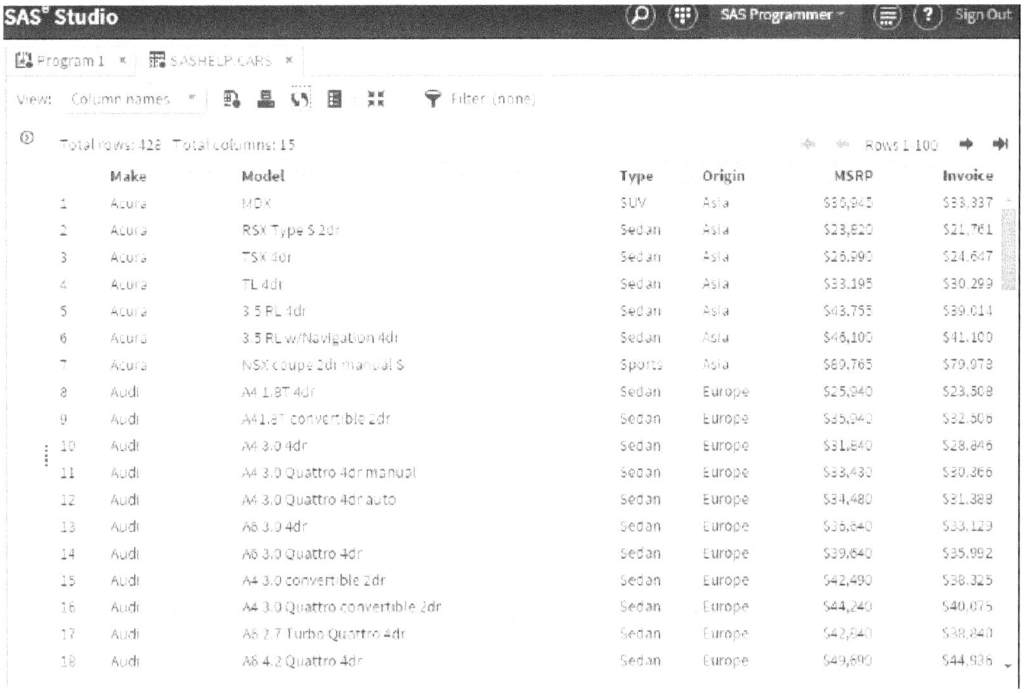

You can right-click a column heading to filter and sort the data table by that column. Right-click the **Invoice** column and select **Add Filter**. Notice that the other options are Sort Ascending, Sort Descending, and Sort by Data Order.

Add a filter to select only the rows with Invoice values greater than or equal to $30,000. Use the drop-down menu to change the filter in the Add Filter window shown in Figure 1.6. Add the filter value in the text box. Then click **Filter**.

**Figure 1.6: Add Filter Window**

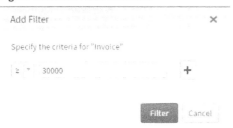

At the top of the table, you see that the number of filtered rows is 160.

As you select options and customize the table, SAS Studio generates SAS code that you can use. To view the query code, click the **Display Query** button on the toolbar.

A new Program tab is created with the code that is used to create the view of the table. This code first creates a new data table in the **Work** library and then prints the data table. You can save this code for use later with the Save button on the toolbar. Close the Query code. Exit the maximized view and expand the **Columns** pane to get back to the default table view. You can clear the table filter by selecting **Clear Filter** on the Tools table.

## Accessing Data in SAS Libraries

SAS tables are stored in SAS libraries. A SAS library is a collection of SAS files that are referenced and stored as a unit. Each file is a member of the library. **Work** is a temporary library where you can store and access SAS tables for the duration of the SAS session. It is the default library.

> **Note:** SAS deletes the **Work** library and its contents when the SAS session ends.

**Sashelp** is a permanent library that contains sample SAS tables that you can access during your SAS session. **Sasuser** is a permanent library that you can use to store and access SAS tables in any SAS session.

Users can create their own SAS libraries.

- A user-defined library is permanent. Tables are stored until the user deletes them.
- A user-defined library is implemented within the operating environment's file system.
- It is not automatically available in a SAS session.

### Accessing a Permanent Library with the LIBNAME Statement

First, identify the location of the library. For example, a Microsoft Windows folder could be used as a SAS library. You can use an existing folder or create a new one. After a folder is identified or created, the Windows operating system knows about the folder, but SAS does not. To use this folder as a SAS library, you must tell SAS about it. Sometimes this is referred to as making a connection between SAS and the folder.

To connect the folder to SAS, use a SAS LIBNAME statement to associate the libref with the physical location of the folder. The concept of a SAS library is the same regardless of the operating environment, but libraries have different physical implementations depending on the environment. In UNIX and Windows, a library is a directory or folder. On a mainframe, it is an operating system file.

The path must be written in a style appropriate for the environment and should include a full path. Examples are shown below.

- Windows: libname perm 'S:\workshop';
- UNIX: libname perm '~/workshop';
- z/OS: libname perm 'userid.workshop.sasfiles';

The SAS LIBNAME statement is a global SAS statement. It is not required to be in a DATA step or PROC step. It does not require a RUN statement. It executes immediately and remains in effect until changed, canceled, or until the session ends. It uses the following syntax:

```
LIBNAME libref "SAS-library" <options>;
```

The libref must be eight characters or less and begin with a letter or underscore followed by letters, underscores, and digits.

> **Tip:** In the Microsoft Windows environment, an existing folder is used as a SAS library. The LIBNAME statement cannot create a new folder.
>
> In the UNIX environment, an existing directory is used as a SAS library. The LIBNAME statement cannot create a new directory.

In the following example, we are associating the libref SP4R with the folder s:\workshop.

```
libname SP4R "s:\workshop";
```

Check the log after submitting a LIBNAME statement to see that it executed successfully and assigned the libref to the physical folder.

## Data Set Names

As a best practice, refer to **both** the library and the data set in DATA steps and PROC steps by using the convention *library.data-set-name*. To access data in a permanent library, you must use the *library.data-set-name* convention. However, to access the temporary library **Work**, you do not need to use the library name. As a best practice, it is always encouraged to use the library name when you refer to a data set. For example, all of the following data set names are correct:

- SP4R.FROG
- work.cars
- cars

# Writing a Program in SAS Studio

In this section, you will learn how to write a SAS program that enables you to see the cars data in the form of a report. To start a new program, go up to the top bar and click on the circle with seven dots inside and choose **New SAS Program**. You can also press F4 on your keyboard.

In R, we generally pass a data frame matrix or vector to analyze it. In SAS, we are actually going to apply a procedure to a data table.

## Code Editor

In the Program 1 workspace, type the word PROC. As you begin to type, notice the context-sensitive Help, which is useful when you are learning SAS programming, as shown in Figure 1.7.

**Figure 1.7: Context-sensitive Help**

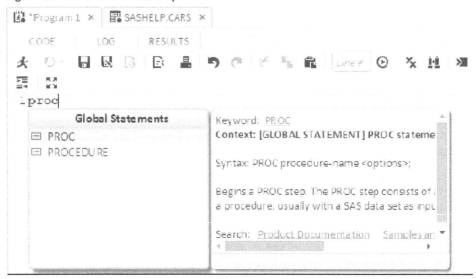

Keep typing and enter the word **print**. Notice how the context-sensitive Help changes. Scroll through the Context Help window. It gives you a little more syntax – BY statements, ID statements, SUM statements, VAR statements. Statements are additional arguments to a procedure. Look at the following syntax for PROC PRINT:

**PROC PRINT** *<option(s)>*;
  **BY** *<DESCENDING> variable-1 <...<DESCENDING> variable-n><NOTSORTED>*;
  **PAGEBY** *BY-variable*;
  **SUMBY** *BY-variable*;
  **ID** *variable(s) <option>*;
  **SUM** *variable(s) <option>*;
  **VAR** *variable(s) <option>*;

The PRINT procedure prints the observations in a SAS data set, using all or some of the variables. You can create a variety of reports ranging from a simple listing to a highly customized report that groups the data and calculates totals and subtotals for numeric variables. Beginning in SAS 9.3, the PRINT procedure is now completely integrated with the Output Delivery System.

The context-sensitive Help also provides links to SAS documentation and samples. To turn off the context Help, in the top bar select **More Application Options ▶ Preferences ▶ Editor**. Clear the **Enable autocomplete** check box. Select **Save**. To view the Context Help without the Autocomplete option, right-click a keyword and select **Syntax Help**.

Finish the program by entering the following code:

```
proc print data=sashelp.cars;
run;
```

This program tells SAS to print the data table **cars** in the **Sashelp** library. The DATA= option tells SAS which data set to use for the specified procedure. Notice that the library name is followed by a period and then the data set name. Notice also that each statement ends with a semicolon.

## Results

By now, you will have noticed that we do not have a command line interpreter. Instead, we are going to compile our code, and the results will be returned.

Print the **cars** data table by clicking **Run** on the toolbar or pressing **F3**. The results are displayed on the RESULTS tab as shown in Figure 1.8.

**Figure 1.8: Program Results**

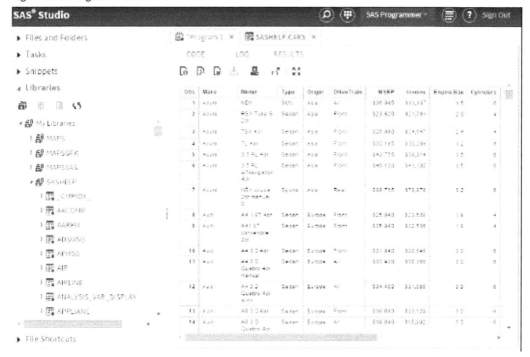

Scroll to view different parts of the table. You can open the results in another window, by clicking the **Open in New Browser** tab. In addition, the toolbar on the Results page provides several ways to save the results. You can download and save the results in a Word, PDF, or HTML document by selecting the appropriate icon.

## Log

As a best practice, always click the **Log** tab to view any errors, warnings, and notes. (See Figure 1.9.)

**Figure 1.9: SAS Log**

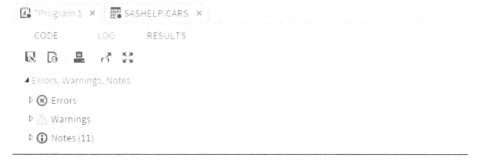

Click the Notes arrow to view the notes that were created. Notice that the log reports that there were 428 observations read from the **sashelp.cars** data set.

> **Tip:** When the log reports errors, it is much easier to click the **Errors** arrow rather than searching for the error throughout the log.

## Adding Variables

Let's create a new program by selecting **New Options** at the top of the page and then selecting **New SAS Program** (or simply press **F4**).

Add the following code to the Program 2 workspace. Use the VAR statement to print only the desired column variables: **Make**, **Model**, **MPG_City**, and **MPG_Highway**.

```
proc print data=sashelp.cars;
    var
run;
```

In the Libraries pane, select the arrow next to the **cars** data set to view the variables in the data set. Drag and drop the four variables into the program after the word var to complete the program. Don't forget to put a semicolon at the end of the statement!

You can see that the names of the variables are capitalized. SAS is not case-sensitive. The variable names could be all-caps, all-lowercase, or any combination of capitalization. This applies to the procedure name and any other part of the syntax.

```
proc print data=sashelp.cars;
    var Make Model MPG_City MPG_Highway;
run;
```

**Tip**: You can also manually enter the name of each variable.

Run the program and view the results, as shown in Figure 1.10. Notice that only the four variables specified in the VAR statement are printed on the Results page.

**Figure 1.10: Program Results**

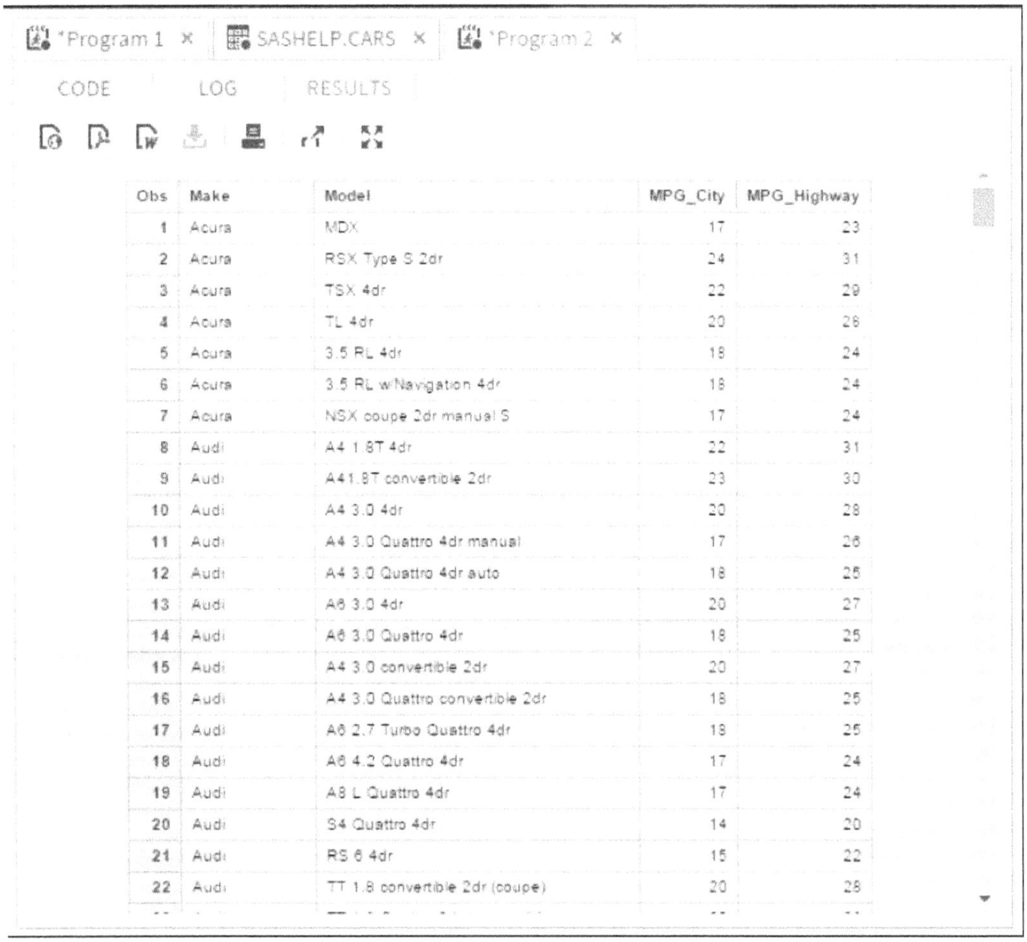


| Obs | Make | Model | MPG_City | MPG_Highway |
|---|---|---|---|---|
| 1 | Acura | MDX | 17 | 23 |
| 2 | Acura | RSX Type S 2dr | 24 | 31 |
| 3 | Acura | TSX 4dr | 22 | 29 |
| 4 | Acura | TL 4dr | 20 | 28 |
| 5 | Acura | 3.5 RL 4dr | 18 | 24 |
| 6 | Acura | 3.5 RL w/Navigation 4dr | 18 | 24 |
| 7 | Acura | NSX coupe 2dr manual S | 17 | 24 |
| 8 | Audi | A4 1.8T 4dr | 22 | 31 |
| 9 | Audi | A41.8T convertible 2dr | 23 | 30 |
| 10 | Audi | A4 3.0 4dr | 20 | 28 |
| 11 | Audi | A4 3.0 Quattro 4dr manual | 17 | 26 |
| 12 | Audi | A4 3.0 Quattro 4dr auto | 18 | 25 |
| 13 | Audi | A6 3.0 4dr | 20 | 27 |
| 14 | Audi | A6 3.0 Quattro 4dr | 18 | 25 |
| 15 | Audi | A4 3.0 convertible 2dr | 20 | 27 |
| 16 | Audi | A4 3.0 Quattro convertible 2dr | 18 | 25 |
| 17 | Audi | A6 2.7 Turbo Quattro 4dr | 18 | 25 |
| 18 | Audi | A6 4.2 Quattro 4dr | 17 | 24 |
| 19 | Audi | A8 L Quattro 4dr | 17 | 24 |
| 20 | Audi | S4 Quattro 4dr | 14 | 20 |
| 21 | Audi | RS 6 4dr | 15 | 22 |
| 22 | Audi | TT 1.8 convertible 2dr (coupe) | 20 | 28 |

## Using Tasks

In addition to features that make writing SAS code easier, SAS Studio also includes powerful point-and-click tasks that quickly generate reports and graphs. Let's learn how to use tasks to generate summary statistics and plots.

To see all available tasks, select **Tasks** in the Navigation pane and then expand **Tasks** (Figure 1.11).

**Figure 1.11: Tasks**

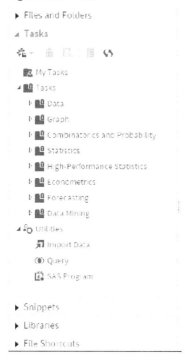

Notice that the tasks are separated into the following categories based on the analysis:

- Data
- Graph
- Combinatorics and Probability
- Statistics
- High-Performance Statistics
- Econometrics
- Forecasting
- Data Mining

You can expand each node to view the possible tasks. Expand the **Statistics** task and double-click the **Summary Statistics** task. Notice that a new tab with some initialized code opens with the title Summary Statistics, as shown in Figure 1.12. All of the text in green (just like in R) is comment code. Everything between the /* and the */ is going to be commented out.

**Figure 1.12: Summary Statistics Task**

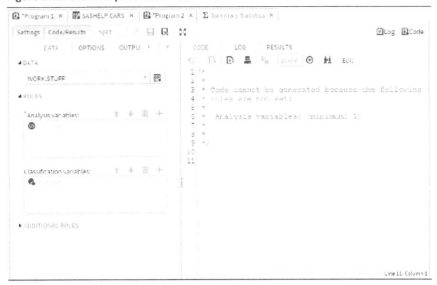

In the Data section, click the **Select a Table** button and navigate to the **cars** data set in the **Sashelp** library. Click the **plus** symbol next to Analysis variables and select **Weight** as the analysis variable. Notice that SAS Studio automatically generates the code for the MEANS procedure, as shown in Figure 1.13.

**Figure 1.13: Summary Statistics Task—Data Section**

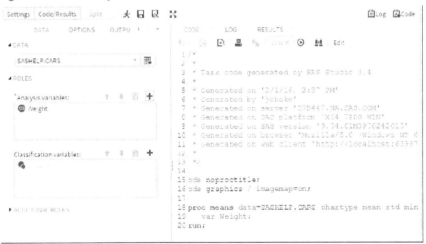

Click the **OPTIONS** tab to specify which options you want to use. Ignore the Basic Statistics options. In the Plots section, select the **Histogram** and **Add normal density curve** check boxes to create statistical graphics. Again, notice that SAS Studio automatically generates the code for the additional options, as shown in Figure 1.14.

**Figure 1.14: Summary Statistics Task—Options Section**

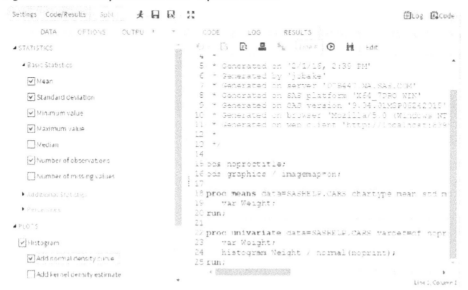

Run the generated code and view the results. The analysis is shown in a summary table and the plot is also printed on the Results page (Figure 1.15).

**Figure 1.15: Summary Statistics Task—Results**

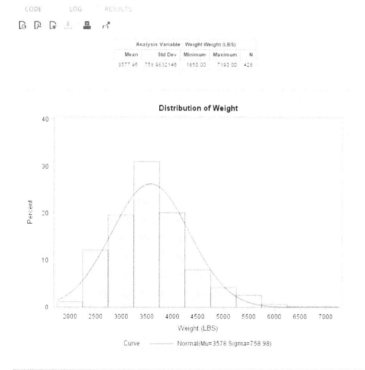

---

**Tip**: You can save the program by clicking the **Save** button on the toolbar or by copying and pasting the code into an existing program.

---

## Using Snippets

Code snippets enable you to quickly insert saved SAS code in your program and customize the code to meet your needs. Think of snippets as starter code. If there is code that you run often that you don't want to have to type in every time from scratch, save it as a snippet. Let's use snippets to create a scatterplot matrix.

## Preloaded Snippets

Open a new program tab by pressing **F4**. In the Navigation pane, select **Snippets** and then expand the **Snippets** arrow. In Figure 1.16 you can see the preloaded snippet categories.

Figure 1.16: Snippets

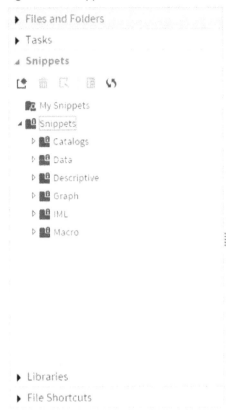

Expand **Graph**. Drag and drop the **Scatter Plot Matrix** snippet into the program workspace. The following code is generated:

```
/*--Scatter Plot Matrix--*/
title 'Vehicle Profile';
proc sgscatter data=sashelp.cars(where=(type in ('Sedan' 'Sports')));
    label mpg_city='City';
    label mpg_highway='Highway';
    matrix mpg_city mpg_highway horsepower weight /
       transparency=0.8 markerattrs=graphdata3(symbol=circlefilled);
run;
```

This code will open up every time you click this snippet. It will not change. Notice that we are working with the sashelp.cars data. This is a complete coincidence! Click **Run** and view the results. (See Figure 1.17.)

**Figure 1.17: Snippet Code Results**

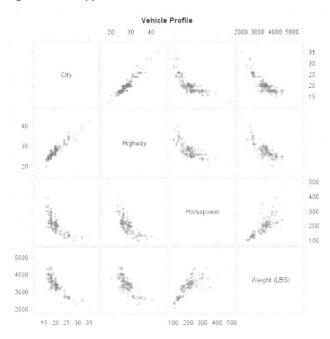

> **Tip**: Generally, snippets are used as a starter program. Thus, the generated code can be altered to fit your needs.

Let's go back to the code because, remember, snippets are just started code. Delete the WHERE option and change the **Weight** variable to the **Length** variable to create the following code:

```
/*--Scatter Plot Matrix--*/
title 'Vehicle Profile';
proc sgscatter data=sashelp.cars;
    label mpg_city='City';
    label mpg_highway='Highway';
    matrix mpg_city mpg_highway horsepower length /
      transparency=0.8 markerattrs=graphdata3(symbol=circlefilled);
run;
```

Click **Run** and view the results from the modified snippet (Figure 1.18).

**Figure 1.18: Modified Snippet Code Results**

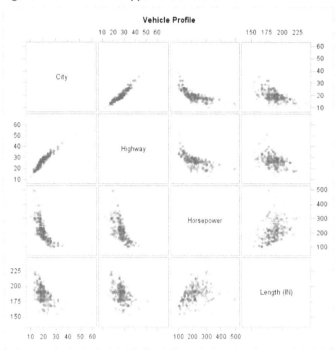

### Custom Snippets

Create your own snippet by clicking the **New Snippet** button in the Snippets pane. Copy and paste the SAS code that you want to use onto the Snippet 1 tab. Click **Save** on the Snippet 1 tab. In the Add to My Snippets window, type a name for your Snippet and click **Save**.

Notice that the My Snippets section now has your custom snippet, which you can drag and drop onto any SAS Studio Program tab at your convenience.

## Calling R from SAS

In this section, you will see how easy it is to work with R from SAS/IML. We can export our data to R and write R code directly in IML. This section includes advanced programs and techniques that show you what you will be able to do by the end of this book. We will not talk through the details of the code, but rather this will just show you what we are working toward at the end of this book.

For this example, we will use the randomForest package in R. We will send the **birth** data set to R, use the randomForest() function to create a predictive model, and return the results to SAS.

Program 1.2 invokes SAS/IML and sends the birth data set in the Work library to R and names the data frame birth as well. Write your R code between the SUBMIT and ENDSUBMIT statements. Use the randomForest package in R and the randomForest() function to estimate a model with **BWT** as the dependent variable and **Smoke, HT, LWT**, and **PTL** as independent variables. Use the SUMMARY statement to print the details of the analysis to the console. Finally, create a data frame with the actual and predicted values, given the model, and name the variables **Actual** and **Predicted**.

**Program 1.2: RandomForest Function**

```
proc iml;
    call ExportDataSetToR("work.birth","birth");

submit / r;
    library(randomForest)
    rf = randomForest(BWT ~ SMOKE + HT + LWT + PTL,
      data=birth,ntree=200,importance=TRUE)
    summary(rf)
```

```
    actual = birth$BWT
    pred = predict(rf,data=birth)
    actual.pred = cbind(actual,pred)
    colnames(actual.pred) <- c("Actual","Predicted")
endsubmit;

    call ImportDataSetFromR("Rdata","actual.pred");
quit;
```

Remember that we returned our data set, which opens in a new tab in OUTPUT DATA. Return the data frame to a SAS data set with the name **Rdata**.

> **Tip:** The output from the Summary function generated in the R console was printed in the SAS Results page as shown in Output 1.2. By default, SAS returns all the R console output directly to the SAS Results page, keeping it in R format.

**Output 1.2: Results from Program 1.2**

|  | Length | Class | Mode |
| --- | --- | --- | --- |
| call | 5 | -none- | call |
| type | 1 | -none- | character |
| predicted | 189 | -none- | numeric |
| mse | 200 | -none- | numeric |
| rsq | 200 | -none- | numeric |
| oob.times | 189 | -none- | numeric |
| importance | 8 | -none- | numeric |
| importanceSD | 4 | -none- | numeric |
| localImportance | 0 | -none- | NULL |
| proximity | 0 | -none- | NULL |
| ntree | 1 | -none- | numeric |
| mtry | 1 | -none- | numeric |
| forest | 11 | -none- | list |
| coefs | 0 | -none- | NULL |
| y | 189 | -none- | numeric |
| test | 0 | -none- | NULL |
| inbag | 0 | -none- | NULL |
| terms | 3 | terms | call |

> **Tip:** If you are running SAS Studio in client/server mode, you do **not** have access to the **Work** library on a point-and-click basis. You must use the PRINT procedure to view the results.

# Exercises

1. Choose the correct statement.

   a. SAS has a command line interpreter.

   b. SAS is case sensitive.

   c. SAS Studio and SAS University Edition are synonymous.

   d. SAS applies procedures to the data table for analysis.

2. Which statement is a SAS syntax requirement?

   a. Begin each statement in column one.

   b. Put only one statement on each line.

   c. Separate each step with a line space.

   d. End each statement with a semicolon.

1. How many statements are contained this DATA step?

```
data work.newsalesemps;
    length First_Name $ 12 Last_Name $ 18 Job_Title $ 25;
    infile "&path\newemps.csv" dlm=',';
    input First_Name $ Last_Name $
    Job_Title $ Salary;
run;
```

# Solutions

## Multiple Choice

1. d
2. d

## Short Answer

1. This DATA step has five statements.

# Chapter 2: Importing and Reporting Data

## Introduction

Now that you are comfortable navigating SAS Studio and have a feel for SAS syntax, in this chapter we will learn how to import data into SAS. We will start by creating a few data sets manually with the DATA step and then we will import some delimited raw data files. After we create new SAS data sets, you will learn how to report different features of the data, including how to change the appearance of SAS column headings and values with SAS labels and formats.

For the rest of this book, you will generally see a "Duplicate the R Script" step. We will look at how to do something in R and then show how to do it in SAS.

## Manual Data Entry with the DATA Step

In this section, we want to create a data set by hand. For example, suppose we want to create a data set with 4 variables: first name, last name, age, and height. These variables are a mix of character and numeric values.

### Create a New Data Set

To create a new SAS data set, we are going to use a DATA step. Recall from Chapter 1 that DATA steps are used to read in data or alter existing data sets. In SAS, the syntax of the DATA step is:

```
DATA new-data-set-name;
   LENGTH variable-a <$> # variable-a <$> # ...;
   INPUT variable-a<$>    variable-b   ...;
   DATALINES;
   a1 b1 ... z1
   a2 b2 ... z2
   ...
```

```
an bn ... zn
  ;
run;
```

> **Tip:** The < > symbols denote optional SAS syntax.

We start with the DATA statement and specify a new data set name, and then we use the input statement to specify the variables to be in the data set. If the variables are character values, we need to specify a dollar sign after the variable name.

Next, we specify a data line statement. It is a statement, so we use a semicolon. Then, we start writing our data in columns. So, column 1 is variable a, column 2 is variable b, and so on. After we enter all the data, add a semicolon. Then use a RUN statement to finish up the DATA step.

By default, SAS only gives you 8 bytes in a single variable. Numeric values are stored in floating point notation storing up to 17 significant digits in 8 bytes. In a character variable, each character takes one byte. So by default, they can hold a maximum of 8 characters.

If your data values are longer than 8 characters (for example, names), or shorter than 8 characters (for example, gender or state code), then you can use an optional LENGTH statement to specify a length for the variable. In the LENGTH statement, you can say variable a, then a dollar sign since it's a character variable and then specify a number. How many characters do you want to be able to hold in a single variable? In general, you just need an upper bound. You don't have to go into the data set and identify the largest variable. Maybe you just want to go up to 100 characters. But keep in mind, it's going to save space to have fewer characters. So don't specify a number of bytes that is extremely large because you don't want to save unnecessary space.

> **Tip:** Character variables specified in the LENGTH and INPUT statements must be followed by the $ symbol. However, the INPUT statement does not require the $ symbol if the LENGTH statement is used.

## Example

In R, to create a new data set, we might create 4 vectors (first name, last name, age, and height), and then combine them to create a data frame, as shown in Figure 2.1.

**Figure 2.1: R Script**

```
         Source on Save                              Run     Source
1  First_Name = c("Jordan","Bruce","Walter","Henry","JeanClaude")
2  Last_Name = c("Bakerman","wayne","white","Hill","VanDamme")
3  age = c(27,35,51,65,55)
4  height = c(68,70,70,66,69)
5
6  #Create Data Frame
7  example_data = data.frame(First_Name,Last_Name,age,height)
```

Now let's duplicate the R script in SAS.

**Program 2.1a: Duplicate the R Script in SAS**

```
data sp4r.example_data;
    length First_Name $ 25 Last_Name $ 25;
    input First_Name $ Last_Name $ age height;
    datalines;
    Jordan Bakerman 27 68
    Bruce Wayne 35 70
    Walter White 51 70
    Henry Hill 65 66
    JeanClaude VanDamme 55 69
  ;
run;
```

In Program 2.1a, we are creating a data set called EXAMPLE_DATA and saving it in the SP4R library. In the INPUT statement, there are 4 variables. FIRST_NAME and LAST_NAME are character-valued, so they require dollar signs. AGE and HEIGHT are numeric variables.

Next, we specify the data lines and type in all the data on separate lines. Remember the final semicolon after the data, and don't forget the RUN statement to finish up the DATA statement.

You will notice that the last observation, JeanClaude, has more than 8 bytes. It has 10 characters. So we needed to use a LENGTH statement to change the number of bytes for the variable. In the LENGTH statement, we can specify lengths for FIRST_NAME and LAST_NAME. Here we used 25 characters as a length, but we don't need to know the value with the maximum number of characters if you just specify an upper bound.

Click **Run** to run Program 2.1a to make sure you have created your data set correctly.

In Program 2.1b, we will create another data set. The only difference here is that you will notice we are reading in more than one observation per line.

**Program 2.1b: Duplicate the R Script in SAS Another Way**

```
data sp4r.example_data2;
    length First_Name $ 25 Last_Name $ 25;
    input First_Name $ Last_Name $ age height @@;
    datalines;
    Jordan Bakerman 27 68 Bruce Wayne 35 70 Walter White 51 70
    Henry Hill 65 66 JeanClaude VanDamme 55 69
;
run;
```

In Program 2.1b, we have our first observation and then immediately following it, we have the second and third observations. To read in this data we need to use the trailing @@ symbol in the INPUT statement. That symbol tells SAS to hold the line and continue reading in data as new observations. If we didn't use the trailing @@ symbol, we would only have 2 observations in this data set: Jordan Bakerman and Henry Hill.

> **Tip:** The @@ option at the end of the INPUT statement enables the DATA step to read in more than one observation per line.

## Create a New Data Set with Delimited Data

Let's look at another method for reading in data that uses some of the syntax we just learned, plus some options that will be discussed more in the next section. Perhaps you have a text file and you don't want to import the file, you just want to read in the text values by copying and pasting the data into DATA step. But maybe that text file has delimited data. How can we read that in?

Take a look at Program 2.2 where we create a new data set called EXAMPLE_DATA3.

**Program 2.2: Manually Creating a SAS Data Set from Delimited Data**

```
data sp4r.example_data3;
    length First_Name $ 25;
    infile datalines dlm='*';
    input First_Name $ Last_Name $ age height;
    datalines;
    Jordan*Bakerman*27*68
    Bruce*Wayne*35*70
    Walter*White*51*70
    Henry*Hill*65*66
    Jean Claude*Van Damme*55*69
;
run;
```

In Program 2.2, we use a LENGTH statement to change the first name variable to 25 characters maximum. Notice in this case that we are not setting a length for last name. Our INPUT statement has the same 4 variables: first name, last name, age, and height.

In the DATALINES statement notice that the data is delimited with stars. In order to read in this data, we add an INFILE statement and use the keyword DATALINES. That tells SAS to read in the data under the DATALINES statement, as opposed to a delimited raw data file. We also use the DLM= option, which specifies the delimiter, which in this case is a star.

When you run Program 2.2, the data table created should look exactly like the one created in the previous section. But remember, we only specified a length for the first name field. So the last name field defaults to 8 bytes and some of the data will be truncated.

## Importing Data

In this section, we will learn how to import a saved raw data file using either a DATA step or a PROC step to get back a new SAS data set.

In R, we might use the read.csv function and create new data files from our CSV files. Once we read in the data, then we can use functions like COLNAMES to actually change the data frame column names.

### Import with a DATA Step

To read in a delimited raw data file in SAS, we can use a DATA step. The syntax is very similar to the manual data entry syntax, but you will replace the DATALINES statement with the INFILE statement to read a raw data file as shown below:

**DATA** output-data-set;
  **LENGTH** *variable* <$> # **variable** <$> #...;
  **INFILE** "*data-file-path*" **DLM=**'*delimiter*'
  **INPUT** *variable* <$> *variable* <$>...;
**RUN;**

Start with the DATA statement, then specify a new SAS data set name. We will use the INPUT statement exactly as before and specify variable names. If the variable is a character data value, use the dollar sign. If we need to change the number of characters to something larger than 8, we will use a LENGTH statement.

This time, however, instead of using the DATALINES statement, we will use the INFILE statement. In quotation marks, specify the path to the file. For example, an INFILE statement might look like the following:

```
infile "&path/example.csv";
```

The INFILE statement identifies the raw data file to be read and requires the delimiter option, DLM, if the raw data file is separated by something other than a space. For example, if your data is comma-delimited, your INFILE statement might look like the following:

```
infile "&path\allnames.csv" dlm=',';
```

The INFILE statement must come before the INPUT statement. Some common delimiters are DLM=',' for .csv and DLM='09'x for tab-delimited files.

### Import with PROC IMPORT

An alternative method to reading in delimited raw data files is the IMPORT procedure. The DATA step requires a bit more syntax, but gives you more control over how exactly to read in delimited raw data files. PROC IMPORT is a helpful method for use with files with more structure like CSV files or Excel workbooks. For example, if the first row in the data file has the variable names that you want to use in the SAS data set, PROC IMPORT makes it very easy to use those as the SAS variable names.

For the PROC IMPORT procedure, the syntax to import a file with column names is below:

**PROC IMPORT OUT=**data-set-name
  **DATAFILE=** "*data-file-path*"
  **DBMS=**identifier <REPLACE>;

```
     GETNAMES=<yes,no>;
     SHEET=<"sheet.name">
     DATAROW=<#>;
RUN;
```

Start with a PROC IMPORT statement. In the OUT= option, you will specify the new SAS data set name. The next option, the DATAFILE= option lets you specify the full path to the data file (similar to the INFILE statement before). The DBMS= option is simply the identifier of the file. For example, if you are reading a CSV file, you simply specify CSV. If you are working with an Excel workbook, you would specify xlsx.

If the first row of your data contains the variable names that you want to use as SAS variable names, then use the GETNAMES=yes option to read in those variable names and use them as the SAS data set variable names.

SHEET is a great statement to be aware of. If you are reading in data sets from multiple sheets of an Excel workbook, you can specify the name of the sheet explicitly and read in only that specific data set. You can also specify a data row to start reading in the data. For example, if the first row has column names and the second row is blank, use DATAROW=3.

> **Tip:** The REPLACE option is used to write over existing SAS data tables with the same name.

If you read in a delimited raw data file with PROC IMPORT and you don't have variable names that you are going to use as SAS data set variable names, the variable names will default to var1, var2, var3, and so on. To change those after the data has been read in, you'll need to use the DATA step. Simply specify the name of the data set we are working with and the SET statement tells SAS where to pull the data from. If the data set names and the data in the set statements are the same, it simply writes over that data set with our changes.

You can change as many variable names in a single RENAME statement as you want. To rename the variables, use the RENAME statement as shown below:

```
DATA data-table-name-new;
   SET data-table-name-old;
      RENAME     old-var-1= new-var-1
                 old-var-2= new-var-2
                 …
                 old-var-n= new-var-n;
RUN;
```

## Examples

Figure 2.2 shows an instance of reading in a CSV file in R. In this example, we will read in a delimited raw data file with a DATA step to duplicate the results from the R script in Figure 2.2.

**Figure 2.2: R Script**

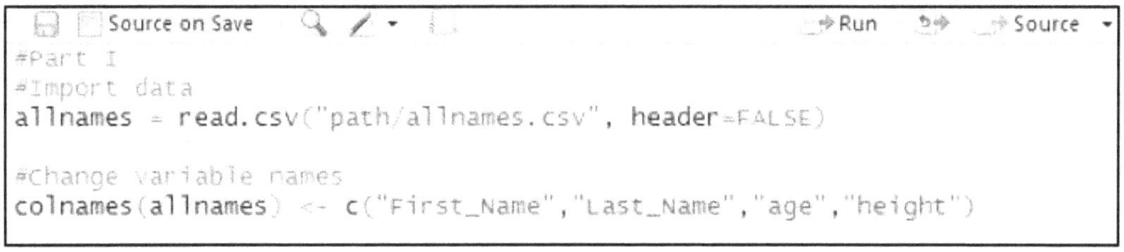

In Program 2.3 we are printing a new data set called ALL_NAMES in the SP4R library. The allnames.csv file has the original five names that were used in the previous example as well as 195 other names. Of course, we would not want to type those out by hand! It's much easier to save them in a CSV file and read them in with a DATA step.

**Program 2.3: Duplicate the R Script with a DATA Step**

```
data sp4r.all_names;
    length First_Name $ 25 Last_Name $ 25;
```

```
    infile "&path\allnames.csv" dlm=',';
    input First_Name $ Last_Name $ age height;
run;
```

The variable names are going to be the same names as in the example in the previous section: First_Name, Last_Name, age, and height. In the LENGTH statement in Program 2.3, we change the length of the first name and last name variables. In the INFILE statement, we specify the path to the data file. With the DLM= option, we specify the comma as the delimiter for the CSV file type. If you run this program, you should see a table with 200 observations in 4 columns.

Figure 2.3 shows an instance of reading in a CSV file in R. In this example, we will read in a delimited raw data file with a PROC step to duplicate the results from the R script in Figure 2.3.

**Figure 2.3: R Script**

```
#Part II
#Import data with variable names
baseball = read.csv("path/baseball.csv")

#Change variable names
colnames(baseball) <- c("Name","Team","At_Bats","Hits","Home_Runs",
                        "Runs","RBIs","League","Division",
                        "Position","Errors")
```

To duplicate this R script in SAS, let's import a data set with the IMPORT procedure as shown in Program 2.4.

**Program 2.4: Duplicate the R Script with PROC IMPORT**

```
proc import out=sp4r.baseball
    datafile= "&path\baseball.csv" DBMS=CSV REPLACE;
    getnames=yes;
    datarow=2;
run;

data sp4r.baseball;
    set sp4r.baseball;
    rename     nAtBat = At_Bats
               nHits = Hits
               nHome = Home_Runs
               nRuns = Runs
               nRBI = RBIs
               nError = Errors;
run;
```

In the PROC IMPORT statement, we use the OUT= option to specify the data set name. In the DATAFILE= option, we specify the path to the baseball.csv data file. The file type is, of course, CSV. We use the REPLACE option to overwrite any existing data sets in the SP4R library with the same name.

Now this CSV has the first row with the variable names that we want to use as SAS data set variable names, so we use the GETNAMES=yes option. Then we tell SAS to start reading in the data on row 2.

Run just the IMPORT procedure portion of Program 2.4 by highlighting only that portion of the code. In the OUTPUT DATA tab, we can see the data set, which is from the 1986 MLB season. It includes the names of players, the team that they played for, and several other variables indicating player performance. You will notice that the performance measure variable names start with n: nAtBat, nHits, nHome, and so on. Maybe we don't the n character in front of all those variable names.

To change the variable names, we use the RENAME statement in a DATA step, as shown in the second part of the code in Program 2.4. In the DATA statement and the SET statement, we specify the same name, baseball. This overwrites the existing data set. In the RENAME statement, we change nAtBat to At_Bats, nHits to Hits, and so on. Once you run the second part of the code in Program 2.4, your data set will display with the new variable names.

# Reporting Data

Now that we know how to get our data into SAS, we want to report the data and bring some features into a report. To do this, we will use a few different PROC steps and return some results.

In R, when we read in a data set, we can use several different functions including:

- head() to print the first 6 rows to make sure we read it in correctly
- names() to see the variable names
- dim() to see the dimension of the data set
- levels() to identify the unique levels of the classification variables

In R, we can also print variables conditionally. We can do all this in SAS with a few different procedures.

## PROC CONTENTS

The first reporting procedure that we will learn about is the CONTENTS procedure. It provides the same information as the R functions dim() and names(). It provides us the number of observations, the number of variables, as well as the variable names in the data set. Program 2.5 shows a simple CONTENTS procedures and Output 2.5 shows the results of running the program.

**Program 2.5: CONTENTS Procedure**

```
proc contents data=sp4r.cars varnum;
run;
```

**Output 2.5: Results of Program 2.5**

| Data Set Name | WORK.CARS | Observations | 428 |
|---|---|---|---|
| Member Type | DATA | Variables | 23 |

Variables in Creation Order

| # | Variable | Type | Len | Format | Label |
|---|---|---|---|---|---|
| 1 | mpg_quality | Char | 6 | | |
| 2 | Make | Char | 13 | | |
| 3 | Model | Char | 40 | | |

As a best practice, use the VARNUM option in the CONTENTS statement so that SAS will print the variables to the results page in the order in which they appear in the data set. Of course, in SAS Studio, if you wanted to, you could simply open up your data set and view that information in the appropriate data table tab.

## PROC PRINT

### FIRSTOBS= and OBS= Options

To reproduce the head() function in R, we simply use the FIRSTOBS= and the OBS= option in the PROC PRINT statement. As shown in Program 2.6, in parentheses, we will say FIRSTOBS=1 and OBS=6, which will print just observations 1 through 6, as shown in Output 2.6.

**Program 2.6: FIRSTOBS= and OBS= Options in Print Procedure**

```
proc print data=sp4r.cars (firstobs=1 obs=6);
run;
```

**Output 2.6: Results of Program 2.6**

| Obs | mpg_quality | Make | Model | Type | Origin | DriveTrain | MSRP | Invoice |
|-----|------------|------|-------|------|--------|-----------|------|---------|
| 1 | Medium | Acura | MDX | SUV | Asia | All | $36,945 | $33,337 |
| 2 | Medium | Acura | RSX Type S 2dr | Sedan | Asia | Front | $23,820 | $21,761 |
| 3 | Medium | Acura | TSX 4dr | Sedan | Asia | Front | $26,990 | $24,647 |
| 4 | Medium | Acura | TL 4dr | Sedan | Asia | Front | $33,195 | $30,299 |
| 5 | Medium | Acura | 3.5 RL 4dr | Sedan | Asia | Front | $43,755 | $39,014 |
| 6 | Medium | Acura | 3.5 RL w/Navigation 4dr | Sedan | Asia | Front | $46,100 | $41,100 |

Of course, you can change the numbers in the FIRSTOBS= and OBS= options. If you wanted to print observations 10 through 20, you could simply change those options as you see fit. By default, PROC PRINT displays all observations and all variables if you do not use the OBS= option.

> **Tip:** If you start from observation 1, you do not need FIRSTOBS=1.

### WHERE Statement

We saw in Chapter 1 that to print only specified variable, we simply list them in the VAR statement. But what if we wanted to print observations conditionally? We can use a WHERE statement and provide it a conditional expression, as shown in the syntax below:

```
PROC PRINT DATA=data-table <options>;
   VAR variable1 variable2 …;
   WHERE conditional-expression;
RUN;
```

The WHERE statement is very powerful and consistent. It can be used in other procedures as well. Here are some examples of WHERE expressions:

- where salary > 5000
- where gender='Male';
- where upcase(gender)='MALE';

The last two examples show one of the few instances where SAS is case-sensitive. Notice that we are quoting the word 'Male'. In that case, you need to specify the observations exactly as it appears in the SAS data table. If it appears as Male, you need to specify it exactly that way. It will not find observations for 'male'. To avoid case sensitivity, you can use the UPCASE function to capitalize all observations.

### PROC SQL

To reproduce the levels() function in R to actually find the unique levels of a classification variable, we will use PROC SQL (pronounced "sequel"). PROC SQL is a very large, very powerful procedure that can do lots of different tasks. For example, it can subset data, call data, and combine data. Any type of querying of data can be done using PROC SQL. If you are familiar with the open-source SQL, you can use all the same functionality directly in SAS. The only difference is that you have to use the PROC SQL step.

To print the unique levels of a classification variable, the PROC SQL syntax is shown below.

**PROC SQL;**
   **SELECT UNIQUE** *variable-name* **FROM** *data-table-name*;
**QUIT;**

Use the SELECT UNIQUE statement and then specify the variable name for which you want to print unique levels. Use the keyword FROM and specify the data table to be queried.

In Program 2.7, we query the CARS database to select the unique levels of the variable ORIGIN.

**Program 2.7: PROC SQL**

```
proc sql;
    select unique origin from sp4r.cars;
quit;
```

**Output 2.7: Results of Program 2.7**

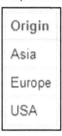

| Origin |
| --- |
| Asia |
| Europe |
| USA |

In Output 2.7, you can see that it prints Asia, Europe, and USA.

## Comparison Operators

Most of the comparison operators in SAS are exactly the same as in R. Greater than, less than, greater than or equal to, and less than or equal to are exactly the same. The ones that are different are the equal to and not equal to operators. In SAS, we do not use the exclamation point to denote not equal to something, but we do have three other options as shown in Table 2.1. Also, we do not use the double equal sign in SAS. If you are using multiple equal signs in SAS, the first equal sign is actually the assignment and the second equal sign acts as the binary operator.

**Table 2.1: Comparison Operators**

| R operator | SAS operator | Mnemonic | Definition |
| --- | --- | --- | --- |
| == | = | EQ | Equal to |
| != | ^= ¬= ~= | NE | Not equal to |
| > | > | GT | Greater than |
| < | < | LT | Less than |
| >= | >= | GE | Greater than or equal to |
| <= | <= | LE | Less than or equal to |
| OR | | IN | Equal to one of a list |

You can also use the mnemonic terms listed in Table 2.1 if you don't want to write out the symbols or cannot remember the symbols in SAS.

Another really powerful operator is the IN operator. This asks the question, "Is it equal to one of a list?" It's very similar to the OR operator in R.

As an example, suppose we want to print observations where country is in the following list:

```
where country in ('US', 'CA');
```

We use parentheses and specify the list: US, Canada. Again, if it's quoted, it's case-sensitive. So in a PROC PRINT statement, this WHERE statement is only going to print observations where the country is either US or Canada.

The logical operators AND and OR have the symbols in SAS as they do in R, as shown in Table 2.2. Again, the exclamation point is not used in SAS, so you have to use one of the three symbols that are acceptable.

Table 2.2: Logical Operators

| R operator | SAS operator | Mnemonic | Priority |
|------------|--------------|----------|----------|
| ! | ^ ¬ ~ | NOT | I |
| & | & | AND | II |
| \| | \| | OR | III |

You can also just use the mnemonic terms NOT, AND, or OR.

As another example, suppose we want to print observations where the country is not either the US or Canada. We would use the following operators in the WHERE statement:

```
where country not in ('US', 'CA');
```

# Enhanced Reporting

In this section we will apply labels and formats to our data sets and results to alter the presentation of the data table or report. We will learn how to change the display of column and variable names, apply formats such as dollar signs to numeric variables, and change date formats.

## LABEL Statement

The LABEL statement is used to change the display of the column variables. The syntax is as follows:

**LABEL** variable-1='label-1' … variable-n='label-n'**;**

In the LABEL statement, we specify the variable name then set it equal to a new variable name. Program 2.8 shows an example of how to change the column names from FN and LN to First Name and Last Name.

**Program 2.8: LABEL Statement**
```
proc print data=sp4r.business label;
    label FN='First Name' LN='Last Name'
run;
```

In the LABEL statement, we specify the variable name FN and set it equal to a new display – "First Name". We do the same thing for LN and set it equal to "Last Name". This only changes the *display* of the columns. The variable names remain FN and LN.

When you are using a LABEL statement with a PRINT procedure, you have to use the LABEL option. But in other procedures, you can just use the LABEL statement.

## Format Statement

Next, let's learn how to apply formats. Formats change the appearance of the observations in a report. They do not change the actual value.

Here are few examples of using formats to change the appearance of observations:

- 10866 (SAS Date) → 01/10/1989
- 5950.35 → $5,950.35

All SAS formats have the following syntax:

<$>*format*<w>.<d>

| | |
|---|---|
| $ | Optional. Indicates a character format. |
| *format* | Names the SAS format. |
| *w* | Optional. Specifies the total format width, including decimal places and special characters. |
| . | Required syntax. Formats always contain a period (.) as part of the name. |
| *d* | Optional. Specifies the number of decimal places to display in numeric formats. |

Formats begin with a $ if it is a character format, followed by the name of the format, an optional width, and a required dot delimiter. The format also contains an optional number of decimal places for numeric formats.

SAS has many built-in character, numeric, data and time, and ISO 8601 formats. An extensive list of these formats can be found on the following page:
http://support.sas.com/documentation/cdl/en/leforinforref/64790/HTML/default/viewer.htm#p0z62k899n6a7wn1r5in6q5253v1.htm

So how do we actually apply a format? Program 2.9 shows an example of using a format statement in a PRINT procedure.

**Program 2.9: FORMAT Statement**
```
proc print data=sp4r.business;
    format salary dollar8. hire_date mmddyy10.;
run;
```

In the PRINT procedure, we specify the variable in the data set in the FORMAT statement. Then, immediately following the variable name (SALARY), we specify the format to be applied to the variable (DOLLAR8). Then we apply the format MMDDYY10 to the variable HIRE_DATE.

As you can see in Output 2.9, Salary now has a dollar sign and a comma and Hire_Date is in a readable date format.

**Output 2.9: Results of Program 2.9**

| Salary | Hire_Date |
|--------|-----------|
| $51,500 | 06/01/1993 |
| $83,975 | 01/01/1978 |
| $94,545 | 04/07/1975 |

**Tip:** As a best practice, use LABEL and FORMAT statements directly in the DATA step when you are reading in your data. When you do this, it automatically applies these labels and formats going forward. If you open up your data set, you will actually see the labels and formats already applied.

If you create a report, it will apply those labels and formats also. That way, you don't have to explicitly specify LABEL and FORMAT statements going forward.

## Formats

Let's look at an example of some common formats. The middle column of Table 2.3 is the stored value in the SAS data set.

**Table 2.3: SAS Format Examples**

| Format | Stored Value | Displayed Value |
|--------|--------------|-----------------|
| DOLLAR12.2 | 27134.5864 | $27,134.59 |
| DOLLAR9.2 | 27134.5864 | $27134.59 |
| DOLLAR8.2 | 27134.5864 | 27134.59 |
| DOLLAR5.2 | 27134.5864 | 27135 |
| DOLLAR4.2 | 27134.5864 | 27E3 |

In the first row of Table 2.3, if we apply the DOLLAR12.2 format, it's going to apply the DOLLAR format with a width of up to 12 characters and maximum of 2 decimal places. The width is for all characters and includes the dollar sign, comma, and period. So the displayed value includes 10 characters for this format.

If the format width is not large enough to accommodate a numeric value, the displayed value is automatically adjusted to fit the width. In the second row of the table, we change the width of the format to 9. Notice in the displayed value that the comma is removed. In the third row, when we reduce the width to 8, notice the dollar sign is also removed. When we get to the last value in the table with a width of 4, it is displayed in scientific notation.

## SAS Date Formats

When working with SAS date formats, the value in the data table represents the number of days since January 1, 1960. Thus, a value of zero represents that date. Going forward in time, for example, 366 days forward will represent January 1, 1961. Going even further, 88,399 days represents January 11, 2022. To go back in time prior to January 1, 1960, we will simply use the dash. So -365 represents January 1, 1959, and so on, as shown in Figure 2.4.

**Figure 2.4: SAS Date Format Timeline**

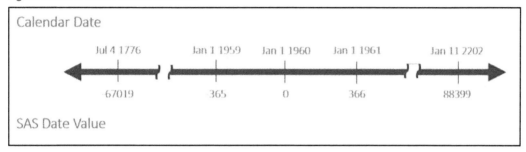

Let's look at an example of how to use SAS date formats. The middle column of Table 2.3 is the stored value in the SAS data set.

**Table 2.4: SAS Date Format Examples**

| Format | Stored Value | Displayed Value |
|--------|--------------|-----------------|
| MMDDYY10. | 0 | 01/01/1960 |
| MMDDYY8. | 0 | 01/01/60 |
| MMDDYY6. | 0 | 010160 |
| DDMMYY10. | 365 | 31/12/1960 |
| DDMMYY8. | 365 | 31/12/60 |
| DDMMYY6. | 365 | 311260 |

If we apply the MMDDYY10 format to a value of zero, it's going to display 01/01/1960. When we reduce the format to the width of 8 to the same value, it simply removes the 19 in the year. When we reduce the width to 6, it removes the slashes. You can see that the width is extremely important when you are displaying a SAS date value.

There are many different formats that you can apply to dates. Table 2.4 shows MMDDYY and DDMMYY formats, which display the order of the day and month differently.

You might be asking yourself, Do I really need to know the number of days since January 1, 1960 to actually work with SAS date formats? The answer, of course, is no. That would be too much of a pain! We use what are called *informats*, meaning that your data is already in the appropriate format. These will be discussed in the example at the end of this section.

## FORMAT Procedure

As mentioned earlier, SAS comes with many built-in formats. However, if SAS does not offer the exact format that you need, you can create your own format.

PROC FORMAT enables you to create your own user-defined formats. To do so, we will use individual value statements and then name the format. The syntax for PROC FORMAT is as follows:

```
PROC FORMAT;
   VALUE <$> format-name range1 = 'label1' …;
RUN;
```

A format name can be a maximum of 32 characters in length. Character formats must begin with a dollar sign followed by a letter or underscore. Numeric formats must begin with a letter or underscore, cannot end in a number, cannot be given the name of a SAS format, and cannot include a period in the VALUE statement.

Labels can be a maximum of 32,767 characters in length and are enclosed in quotation marks.

Let's look at an example of how to use PROC FORMAT to create and apply user-defined format in Program 2.10.

**Program 2.10: PROC FORMAT**

```
proc format;
   value $jobformat  'SR'='Sales Rep'
                     'SM'='Sales Manager';
   value bonusformat 0='No' 1='Yes';
run;

proc print data=sp4r.business;
    format job $jobformat. bonus bonusformat.;
run;
```

In Program 2.10, we create 2 formats in the FORMAT procedure. Recall that if we are working with character data, we start with the dollar sign. We name the first format jobformat. Then we change the display of SR to Sales Rep and SM to Sales Manager.

You can have as many value statements as you want to create as many user-defined formats as you want in a single FORMAT procedure. Next, we create bonusformat, which changes the display of the value 0 to no and 1 to yes. This format can be helpful when working with logistic regression so that you don't have a meaningful response as a value, rather than just a binary 0 or 1.

In the PRINT Procedure, we apply the formats that we have just created to the variables that we want to format. You can see the results of the formats in Output 2.10. Remember that the name of the format must end with a period in the FORMAT statement. After the period is added, the format name becomes green.

**Output 2.10: Results of Program 2.10**

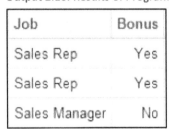

| Job | Bonus |
|---|---|
| Sales Rep | Yes |
| Sales Rep | Yes |
| Sales Manager | No |

> **Tip:** LOW, HIGH, and OTHER are built-in SAS keywords that can be helpful when you format numeric data.

## Example with Informats

In this example, we are creating a data set called EMPLOYEES, as shown in Program 2.11. We have only 2 variables in this data set: Name, a character variable, and Birthday. Notice that for Birthday, we are applying an informat in the first DATA step. To do this, we use the colon to tell SAS that the data we are reading in is already in the specified format. It's already in MMDDYY8.

**Program 2.11: Reporting Example with Informats**

```
data employees;
    input name $ bday :mmddyy8. @@;
    datalines;
    Jill 01011960 Jack 05111988 Joe 08221975
;
run;
```

```
proc print data=employees;
run;
```

If you go to the DATALINES statement, you will see that we have a name and then a date in an MMDDYY format. By using the informat, we don't have to actually calculate the number of days from January 1, 1960. Remember that if you are reading in more than one observation per line, you want to use the trailing @@ symbol.

Run this code to see the results in Output 2.11. Notice that it actually converts the dates to a SAS date value. The bday column is showing the number of days since January 1, 1960.

**Output 2.11: Results of Program 2.11**

| Obs | name | bday |
|-----|------|------|
| 1 | Jill | 0 |
| 2 | Jack | 10358 |
| 3 | Joe | 5712 |

To actually keep the display of labels and formats, let's try this a different way by using the LABEL and FORMAT statements in the DATA step, as shown in Program 2.12. This code is the exact same DATA step as in Program 2.11. The only difference is that now we have a LABEL and FORMAT statements.

**Program 2.12: Reporting Example with Informats, Formats, and Labels**

```
data employees;
    input name $ bday :mmddyy8. @@;
    format bday mmddyy10.;
    label name="First Name" bday="Birthday";
    datalines;
    Jill 01011960 Jack 05111988 Joe 08221975
;
run;

proc print data=employees label;
run;
```

In the first DATA step of Program 2.12, we are reading in the bday variable with the MMDDYY8. format, and then immediately applying a different format, the MMDDYY10. format. We use the LABEL statement to change the display of the column headings. Most SAS procedures apply the stored labels automatically, but remember that PROC PRINT is a little bit different. It only applies labels if you specify the LABEL option in the PROC PRINT statement.

Run this code to see the results in Output 2.12. You will notice the appropriate displays of labels and formats.

**Output 2.12: Results of Program 2.12**

| Obs | First Name | Birthday |
|-----|------------|------------|
| 1 | Jill | 01/01/1960 |
| 2 | Jack | 05/11/1988 |
| 3 | Joe | 08/22/1975 |

# Exercises

Multiple Choice

1. Which DATA step options and statements are missing to correctly read in the **Class** data? (Select all that apply.)

   a.  the @@ option to read in more than one observation per line

   b.  the $ option to read in character data

   c.  the semicolon after the data

   d.  The data set name is case sensitive and should be **CLASS**.

   ```
   data class;
      input grades
      datalines;
      B- A A+ C+ F- A- A B+ B+ B
   run;
   ```

2. Which SAS procedures are used to reproduce the R functions levels(), dim(), head(), and names()?

   a.  PRINT, PRINT, PRINT, CONTENTS

   b.  SQL, CONTENTS, PRINT, CONTENTS

   c.  CONTENTS, PRINT, PRINT, SQL

   d.  SQL, SQL, CONTENTS, PRINT

3. The PROC step below prints the variables **grades**, **student**, and **year** from the **class** data set for all students with grades D or higher. (Assume that the data is clean and there are no + or –grades.)

   ```
   proc print data=class;
       var grades student year;
       where upcase(grades)^='F';
   run;
   ```

   a.  True

   b.  False

Programming Exercise

## 1. Labeling, Formatting, and Conditional Printing

Modify the DATA step, shown below, to complete the exercises. This DATA step generates the CLASS data table with 20 observations and four variables.

```
data sp4r.class;
 input student $ country $ grade bd @@;
 datalines;
 John Spain 95 12000 Mary Spain 82 12121 Alison France 98 12026
 Nadine Spain 77 12222 Josh Italy 61 12095 James France 45 12301
 William France 92 12284 Susan Italy 95 12079
 Charlie France 88 12234 Alice Italy 89 12014 Robert Italy 92 12025
 Emily Spain 87 12148 Arthur Italy 99 12052 Nancy France 70 12238
 Kristin France 65 12084 Sara Italy 49 12322 Ashley Spain 96 12299
 Aaron France 95 12052 Sean France 87 12254 Phil Italy 86 12036
 ;
run;
```

   a.  Use PROC FORMAT to create a format for the GRADE variable.

| Grade | Grade Format |
| --- | --- |
| 0–59 | F |

| 60–69 | D |
| 70–79 | C |
| 80–89 | B |
| 90–100 | A |

b.  Use the DATA step above to read in the Class data set. In the DATA step, label the variable bd as "Birthday" and apply the GradeFormat created in part a. In addition, use the SAS format WORDDATE for the bd variable.

c.  Print the Class data table. (Remember to use the LABEL option in the PRINT statement.)

d.  Use PROC SQL to print the unique levels of the country variable.

e.  Conditionally print the variable student, country, and grade for people with a grade above 79 and from France only.

## Solutions

1. a, b, and c
2. b
3. a

Programming Exercise

1.

a.

```
proc format;
 value gradesformat 0-59='F' 60-69='D' 70-79='C' 80-89='B'
 90-100='A';
run;
```

b.

```
data sp4r.class;
 input student $ country $ grade bd @@;
 label bd='Birthday';
 format grade gradesformat. bd worddate.;
 datalines;
John Spain 95 12000 Mary Spain 82 12121 Alison France 98 12026
Nadine Spain 77 12222 Josh Italy 61 12095 James France 45 12301
William France 92 12284 Susan Italy 95 12079
Charlie France 88 12234 Alice Italy 89 12014 Robert Italy 92 12025
Emily Spain 87 12148 Arthur Italy 99 12052 Nancy France 70 12238
Kristin France 65 12084 Sara Italy 49 12322 Ashley Spain 96 12299
Aaron France 95 12052 Sean France 87 12254 Phil Italy 86 12036
 ;
run;
```

c.

```
proc print data= sp4r.class label;
run;
```

d.

```
proc sql;
 select unique country from sp4r.class;
quit;
```

e.

```
proc print data= sp4r.class;
 var student country grade;
 where grade>79 and country='France';
run;
```

# Chapter 3: Creating New Variables, Functions, and Data Sets

## Introduction

The DATA step is the key to reading your data and altering existing SAS data sets to meet your specifications. In this chapter, we will discuss some additional DATA step techniques for managing day-to-day SAS programming requirements. We will learn how to create and add new variables to an existing SAS data set, use built-in SAS functions to transform data, create new functions, and subset and concatenate SAS data sets.

## Creating New Variables

In this section, you will learn how to create and add new variables to the data set using a DATA step. In R, we typically use the dollar sign syntax to add a variable to our data frame, as seen in Figure 3.1. We will learn how to do the same thing with a DATA step. And by the end of this section, you will learn how to conditionally create a variable using syntax like IF ELSE, IF, and ELSE functions.

**Figure 3.1: R Script**

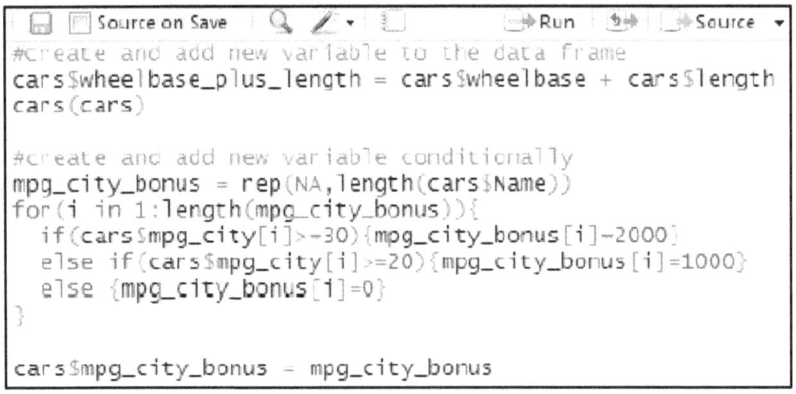

```
[icons] Source on Save    Q  /  -              Run    -    Source  -
#create and add new variable to the data frame
cars$wheelbase_plus_length = cars$wheelbase + cars$length
cars(cars)

#create and add new variable conditionally
mpg_city_bonus = rep(NA,length(cars$Name))
for(i in 1:length(mpg_city_bonus)){
  if(cars$mpg_city[i]>=30){mpg_city_bonus[i]-2000}
  else if(cars$mpg_city[i]>=20){mpg_city_bonus[i]=1000}
  else {mpg_city_bonus[i]=0}
}

cars$mpg_city_bonus - mpg_city_bonus
```

To add a variable to a data set in SAS, we are going to start with our DATA step, specify the name of the data set we're working with, and the same name in the SET statement. Again, this overrides the existing data set with your changes. Recall from Chapter 2 that the syntax of the DATA step is as follows:

**DATA** *new-data-set-name*;
    **LENGTH** *variable-a <$> # variable-a <$> # ...*;
    **INPUT** *variable-a<$>    variable-b  ...*;
    **DATALINES**;
    a1 b1 ... z1
    a2 b2 ... z2
    ...
    an bn ... zn
    ;
**run**;

In Program 3.1, we are creating a new variable called wheelbase_plus_length by adding together two variables in the cars data set. You can add in as many variables as you want in a single DATA step.

**Program 3.1: Duplicate the R Script**

```
data sp4r.cars;
    set sp4r.cars;
    wheelbase_plus_length = wheelbase+length;
run;
```

## Creating Conditional Numeric Variables

Moving on, let's go ahead and create variables conditionally now. Let's tie this to an example. Suppose car manufacturers receive an economic incentive for manufacturing cars with high highway miles per gallon.

Therefore, we want to create a variable called Bonus. We want Bonus to be 2,000 if MPG Highway is greater than or equal to 30 and 1,000 if MPG is between 20 and 29. Otherwise, we want Bonus to be 0.

| MPG Highway | Bonus |
|---|---|
| >=30 | 2,000 |
| 20–29 | 1,000 |
| <20 | 0 |

IF THEN Statements

So how can we accomplish this? We can use IF THEN statements.

> **IF** *expression* **THEN** *statement*;

We will use the cars data set for this example shown in Program 3.2. Using the DATA step, first initialize the new variable, Bonus and set it equal to 2000. This means we are setting every element in the column equal to 2000. Next, use IF statements to change the values conditionally. In the IF statement, we give it an expression. IF *mpg_highway is less than 20* THEN *set bonus equal to 0*. We will use a second IF statement for the last category. IF *mpg_highway is greater than or equal to 20*, AND (the operator that we learned in Chapter 2) *mpg_highway is less than 30,* THEN *set bonus equal to 1000*.

**Program 3.2: Creating a Conditional Variable with the IF THEN Statement**

```
data sp4r.cars;
    set sp4r.cars;
    bonus=2000;
    if mpg_highway<20 then bonus=0;
    if mpg_highway>=20 and mpg_highway<30
    then bonus=1000;
run;
```

> **Tip:** The **bonus = 2000** statement initializes the **bonus** variable.

Using multiple IF statements is not the most efficient way to accomplish this task. Why? Well, because these are mutually exclusive categories. If we test that mpg_highway is less than 20 and we set bonus to 0, we then test another category, which, of course, cannot be possible.

ELSE IF and ELSE Statements

It would be much more efficient if we could fall out of the loop if we tested that the category was true. To do this, we will use the ELSE IF and ELSE statements, just like the ELSE IF and ELSE function in R. The syntax for ELSE IF statements is as follows:

**IF** *expression* **THEN** *statement*;
**<ELSE IF** *expression* **THEN** *statement*;>
<...>
**<ELSE** *statement*;>

In the DATA step in Program 3.3, the first thing you will notice is that the bonus variable has not been initialized. We do not need to do that in SAS. The first IF statement, IF *mpg_highway is less than 20*, THEN, *the first instance of the bonus variable* is set equal to 0. This is the first place we see the bonus variable in this DATA step. Again, we are assuming that Bonus is not in the cars data set in this example.

Next, if the first IF statement is not true, we will go to the next ELSE IF statement. So IF *it is greater than 20* AND *mpg_highway is less than 30*, THEN *bonus equals 1000*. As a catch-all, the ELSE statement sets Bonus equal to 2000. This is much more efficient conditional processing. Again, if we test that the category less than 20 is true, we set bonus equal to 0, fall out of the loop, and don't test any more conditions.

**Program 3.3: Creating a Conditional Variable with ELSE IF and ELSE Statements**

```
data sp4r.cars;
    set sp4r.cars;
    if mpg_highway<20 then bonus=0;
    else if mpg_highway<30 then bonus=1000;
    else bonus=2000;
run;

proc print data=sp4r.cars (firstobs=76 obs=81);
    var mpg_highway bonus;
run;
```

> **Tip:** The **bonus = 1000** statement was removed in favor of the ELSE statement.

Run Program 3.3 and view the results of the PROC PRINT statement to make sure it worked correctly as shown in Output 3.3. If mpg_highway is greater than or equal to 30, we have a bonus of 2000. If it is between 20 and 30, it's a $1,000 bonus. And otherwise, here, mpg_highway at 17 is a bonus of 0.

**Output 3.3: Partial Results of Program 3.3**

| Obs | MPG_Highway | bonus |
|-----|-------------|-------|
| 76  | 32          | 2000  |
| 77  | 30          | 2000  |
| 78  | 28          | 1000  |
| 79  | 32          | 2000  |
| 80  | 28          | 1000  |
| 81  | 17          | 0     |

## Creating Conditional Character Variables

The bonus variable we just created in the previous section was a numeric variable. Now let's create character variables conditionally by looking at another example using the cars data set. Suppose in addition to the Type variable, a variable that indicates whether the vehicle is associated with being a family vehicle should also be in the cars data set.

Let's create a new variable to account for this information in Program 3.4 and call that new variable Type2. If the car type is Hybrid, SUV, Sedan, or Wagon, we will set the Type2 variable to Family Vehicle. Otherwise, we will set the variable to Truck or Sports Vehicle.

| Type | Type2 |
|------|-------|
| Hybrid | Family Vehicle |
| SUV | Family Vehicle |
| Sedan | Family Vehicle |
| Wagon | Family Vehicle |
| Others | Truck or Sports Vehicle |

**Program 3.4: Creating a Conditional Character Variable**

```
data sp4r.cars;
    set sp4r.cars;
    length type2 $ 25; ❶
    if type in ('Hybrid','SUV','Sedan','Wagon') ❷
        then type2='Family Vehicle';
    else type2='Truck or Sports Vehicle'; ❸
run;

proc print data=sp4r.cars (firstobs=61 obs=64);
    var type type2;
run;
```

❶   Remember that any time we are creating new character data, as a best practice, you should use the LENGTH statement. Here we are changing the length of the new character variable type2 (hence, we use the dollar sign), to a maximum of 25 characters.

❷ To create the type2 variable conditionally, first start with the IF statement. IF *type is Hybrid, SUV, Sedan, or Wagon*, THEN *type2 is set to Family Vehicle*.

❸ The catch-all ELSE statement will set type2 equal to Truck or Sports Vehicle.

Looking at the data set in Output 3.4 to make sure it was processed correctly, we can see that the type2 variable is Family Vehicle for Sedan and SUV and Truck or Sports Vehicle for the other two.

**Output 3.4: Results of Program 3.4**

```
Obs    Type       type2

61     Sedan      Family Vehicle
62     Sports     Truck or Sports Vehicle
63     Truck      Truck or Sports Vehicle
64     SUV        Family Vehicle
```

## Creating Conditional Variables with a DO Group

In the previous sections when we used IF, ELSE IF, and ELSE statements, we only executed a single statement after the key word THEN. What if we want to create multiple variables? You will have to execute multiple statements. The way to do this is in SAS is to use a DO group.

The DO group will be used often in the subsequent chapters. We will see it in Chapter 7 when we do matrix simulation and we want to execute something conditionally. It's a great piece of syntax to keep in your back pocket. The general form of conditional DO Group syntax is:

So how do we use the DO group? Well, we begin the same way as an IF THEN statement. IF, specify our expression, THEN we use the keyword DO, followed by a semi-colon. And then we execute whatever statements we want to create as many variables as we want, as shown in the following syntax:

**IF** *expression* **THEN DO;**
  *executable statements*
**END;**
**ELSE IF** *expression* **THEN DO;**
  *executable statements*
**END;**
**ELSE DO;**
  *executable statements*
**END;**

Remember to always end your DO groups with the END statement. The same goes for the ELSE IF and ELSE statements as well!

To practice using the DO group, let's return to our cars data set. Now suppose again that car manufacturers receive an economic incentive for manufacturing cars with high highway miles per gallon. This time, we are going to say that the bonus comes in either one, two, or, if they don't get a bonus, no payments.

If Miles Per Gallon Highway is greater than or equal to 30, we want to create a new variable called Bonus, which is 1,000. And we want to create a new variable called Frequency specifying that they get the bonus in Two Payments. If Miles Per Gallon Highway is between 20 and 29, we will set bonus to 1,000 and say that the frequency comes in only One Payment. And, of course, if they do not receive a bonus, we will just say No Payment for the Frequency variable.

| MPG Highway | Bonus | Frequency |
| --- | --- | --- |
| >=30 | 1,000 | Two Payments |
| 20–29 | 1,000 | One Payment |

| MPG Highway | Bonus | Frequency |
|---|---|---|
| <20 | 0 | No Payment |

To create these two variables conditionally, we will again use a DATA step as shown in Program 3.5.

**Program 3.5: Creating Variables with DO Groups**

```
data sp4r.cars;
    set sp4r.cars;
    length frequency $ 12; ❶
    if mpg_highway<20 then do; ❷
        bonus=0;
        frequency='No Payment';
    end;
    else if mpg_highway<30 then do; ❸
        bonus=1000;
        frequency='One Payment';
    end;
    else do; ❹
        bonus=1000;
        frequency='Two Payments';
    end;
run;

proc print data=cars (firstobs=65 obs=68);
    var mpg_highway frequency;
run;
```

❶  Always remember the LENGTH statement when you are creating character data.

❷  In the first DO group, if miles per gallon highway is less than 20, then we want to do the following: we want to create two variables. Set bonus equal to zero and frequency equal to No Payment. Be sure to use an END statement to end the DO group.

❸  Next, ELSE IF miles per gallon highway is less than 30 and greater than 20, then do the following: set bonus equal to 1,000 and frequency equal to One Payment.

❹  Finally, ELSE do the following: bonus equals 1,000 and frequency equals Two Payments.

When we execute the DATA step and print the data set as shown in Output 3.5, for the first observation we have no bonus and No Payment. The second observation is a bonus of $1,000 and One Payment. And the last observation is a bonus of $1000 and Two Payments.

**Output 3.5: Results of Program 3.5**

```
      MPG_
Obs   Highway    bonus     frequency

65      18         0       No Payment
66      21      1000       One Payment
67      22      1000       One Payment
68      34      1000       Two Payments
```

## Creating and Using Functions

In this section, you will learn how to use some built-in SAS functions to assist in creating new variables—functions like SUM, ABSOLUTE, EXPONENTIATE, ROUND, and so on. We will use all these in a DATA step to create our new variables. By the end of this section, you will have learned how to create your own user-defined function to be used inside a DATA step.

## Creating a Numeric Variable

Figure 3.2 shows a function called mydivision in R with two arguments, numerator and denominator. It returns a value of 0 if the denominator is 0. Otherwise, it returns the value of the numerator divided by denominator.

**Figure 3.2: R Function**

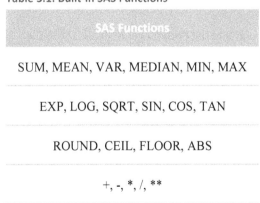

To create a new variable using a built-in SAS function, we will do it the exact same way as in R. In SAS, we will use it in our DATA step using the following syntax:

*new-variable* = FUNCTION(*arguments*);

In Program 3.6, we have our DATA statement, our SET statement, and then we are creating a variable called log_price, which is equal to the log of msrp, meaning we are just taking the log of every element in that variable.

**Program 3.6: SAS Function Example**

```
data sp4r.cars;
    set sp4r.cars;
    log_price = log(msrp);
run;
```

Most functions in SAS operate the exact same way as you would expect coming from R. For example, EXPONENTIATE, LOG, SQUARE ROOT, ROUND, CEILING, FLOOR—they all operate the exact same way, meaning that they apply that operation to every element in the variable.

However, a few of the built-in functions do not operate the way that you would expect coming from R, particularly the first row of Table 3.1—SUM, MEAN, VAR, MEDIAN, MIN, and MAX.

**Table 3.1: Built-in SAS Functions**

| SAS Functions |
| --- |
| SUM, MEAN, VAR, MEDIAN, MIN, MAX |
| EXP, LOG, SQRT, SIN, COS, TAN |
| ROUND, CEIL, FLOOR, ABS |
| +, -, *, /, ** |

> **Note**: SAS does not use the ^ symbol for exponentiation. It uses the double star (**).

When we are using built-in SAS functions in a DATA step, these functions only operate on rows. For example, in R, if we use the SUM function on a vector, it would sum every element of that vector. In SAS, it is only going to apply that operation to each individual row. Applying functions to columns is done using a SAS procedure, which is discussed in Chapter 5.

Let's look at an example to illustrate this in Program 3.7. Here we are creating mean_ miles per gallon, and, using the MEAN function, setting that equal to the mean of miles per gallon highway and miles per gallon city.

**Program 3.7: MEAN Function Example**

```
data sp4r.cars;
  set sp4r.cars;
  mean_mpg = mean(mpg_highway,mpg_city);
run;
```

The function in Program 3.7 is going to the first observation in the cars data set. It's simply taking the mean of those two variables—miles per gallon highway and miles per gallon city—returning the mean, and placing that value in the first row of the new variable, mean miles per gallon. Then it goes to the second row and does the exact same thing. So again, functions only operate on rows in your data set when they are used in a DATA step.

This isn't the best or most efficient way to find some quick summary statistics. A better way is to use a DATA NULL step. Using the key word _NULL_ allows us to avoid creating or altering any SAS data to do some type of operation as shown in Program 3.8.

**Program 3.8: DATA NULL Step**

```
data _NULL_;
    a=mean(1,2,3,4,5);
    b=exp(3);
    c=var(10,20,30);
    d=poisson(1,2);
    put a b c d;
run;
```

In Program 3.8, we are creating the variable a and setting that equal to the mean of the list. b is just equal to e to the third power. c is the variance of 10, 20, and 30. d is the cumulative Poisson distribution with a parameter of 1 and a value of 2.

Because we are not creating a DATA set, if we want to actually see these variables, we have to use the PUT statement. And that just tells SAS to put these to the log so that we can view them, as shown in Output 3.8.

**Output 3.8: Log of Program 3.8**

```
3 20.085536923 100 0.9196986029
```

As you can see in Output 3.8, the mean of those five numbers is 3. e to the third power is about 20.08. The variance of 10, 20, and 30 is 100. And the cumulative distribution function is 0.919.

There are much more efficient ways to actually apply a function to a variable. In Chapter 5, we will talk about some more descriptive procedures to actually find summary statistics that will operate on the entire column or variable. And in Chapter 7, when we get into the interactive matrix language, the functions that we use in there will operate the exact same way coming from R. In IML, when we use the MEAN function, we will actually take the mean of the entire variable.

## Manipulating Character Variables

In the previous section, we were just creating and manipulating numeric data. Let's move on now to manipulating some character values by using built-in functions like SUBSTR, LENGTH, PROPCASE, SCAN, and so on. These will all be used in a DATA step.

Table 3.2 lists just a few of the available built-in functions in SAS and what they can be used to do. There are other functions available, and these can be found in the SAS documentation at support.sas.com/documentation. Click on Programmer's Bookshelf, then under Base SAS, expand the Functions and CALL Routines section to learn more about built-in functions.

Table 3.2: Selected SAS Functions for Character Variables

| SAS Function | Description |
| --- | --- |
| SUBSTR | Extracts a substring from an argument |
| PROPCASE, UPCASE, LOWCASE | Converts word casing |
| SCAN | Returns the nth word from a character string |
| CATX | Removes leading and trailing blanks and concatenates character strings |
| FIND | Searches for the location of a specific substring within a character string |
| TRANWRD | Replaces all occurrences of a substring in a character string |
| PUT | Returns a value using a specified format |

SUBSTR Function

The SUBSTR function allows us to extract a certain part of a string using the following syntax:

*NewVar* = **SUBSTR** (*string, start <,length>*);

If *NewVar* is a new variable, it is created with the same length as the string. To set a different length for *NewVar*, use a LENGTH statement before the assignment statement in the DATA step.

- *String* can be a character constant, variable, or expression.
- *Start* specifies the starting position.
- *Length* specifies the number of characters to extract. If it is omitted, the substring consists of the remainder of *string*.

Imagine you are working with a data set and one of the variables is Acct_Code, as shown below.

| ACCT_Code | Org_Code |
| --- | --- |
| AQI2 | 2 |

We want to create a new variable called Org_Code and just pull out the last character of the Acct_Code variable. we can use the SUBSTR function to do this as shown in the following code:

```
Org_Code = substr(Acct_Code,4,1);
```

Here you can see we are setting Org_Code equal to a SUBSTR function. We pass in the variable, or string—in this case Acct_Code—and then tell SAS to read in characters at the fourth position. We only want to read in one character.

> **Tip:** The SUBSTR function on the left side of an assignment statement is used to replace characters.

LENGTH Function

Now imagine we have multiple observations in the Acct_Code variable. In this case, as shown below, we have three observations, and you will notice they are all different lengths.

| ACCT_Code | Org_Code |
|-----------|----------|
| AQI2 | 2 |
| ES3 | 3 |
| V2 | 2 |

So how can we still pull out that last character? Well, let's just pass the second argument of the SUBSTR function, the LENGTH function, which is the exact same coming from R, as shown in the following syntax:

*NewVar* = **LENGTH** (*argument*);

We pass in the length of the Acct_Code variable, and again just read one character from each string, as shown in the following function:

```
Org_Code=substr(Acct_Code,length(Acct_Code),1);
```

So now our organization code is 2, 3, and 2.

SCAN Function

The SCAN function lets us extract a certain part of a string according to some delimiter using the following syntax:

*NewVar* = **SCAN** (*string, n <,charlist>*);

The SCAN function is used to extract words from a character value when the relative order of words is known, but their starting positions are not. The default delimiter is a blank. When using the SCAN function, the following conditions exist:

- A missing value is returned if there are fewer than *n* words in the string.
- If *n* is negative, the SCAN function selects the word in the character string starting from the end of the string.
- The length of the created variable is the length of the first argument starting in SAS 9.4.
- The length of the created variable is 200 bytes in SAS 9.3 or earlier.
- Delimiters before the first words have no effect.
- Any character or set of characters can serve as a delimiter.
- Two or more contiguous delimiters are treated as a single delimiter.

Suppose we have a data set called Name, which contains the names of employees in a database. The first name in the data set is Farr, Sue, and we want to create a new variable called FName for first name by just pulling out the second word in the name variable.

| Name | FName |
|------|-------|
| Farr,Sue | Sue |

We will do this with the SCAN function as follows:

```
FName = scan(Name,2,',');
```

The function passes the Name variable, or string, specifies what word we are going to be extracting—in this case, the second word—and then the last argument is just the delimiter. The delimiter in this example is a comma. When we execute this statement inside a DATA step, FName is going to be Sue.

### CATX Function

Suppose we want to combine character variables. The CATX function removes leading and trailing blanks, inserts delimiters, and returns a concatenated character string using the following syntax:

*NewVar* = **CATX**(*separator, string-1, … ,string-n*)

Imagine we have a data set with two separate variables—the first name and last name, Sue Farr—and we want to go ahead and concat these two names together and create a new variable called FullName.

| FMName | LName | FullName |
|--------|-------|----------|
| Sue    | Farr  | Sue Farr |

We will use the CATX function as shown below. This also removes leading and trailing blanks so that you don't save any unnecessary space.

```
FullName = catx(' ',FMName,LName);
```

The first argument of the CATX function is just the delimiter. Here we are just giving it a single space. The rest of the arguments in the CATX function are just the strings, or variables, you are going to concatenate together. So here we pass it the variables FMName and LName. The new FullName variable will be Sue space Farr.

### TRANWRD Function

Finally, assume you want to change a certain part of a string or variable and replace it with another string or word. In this case, assume we want to change all instances of the word Luci in the data set below to Lucky in the product variable of our data set.

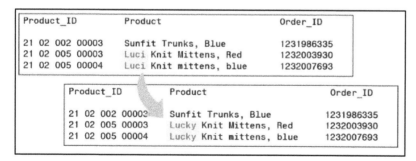

To do this easily, we can use the TRANWRD function with the following syntax:

*NewVar* = **TRANWRD** (*source, target, replacement*);

The TRANWRD function replaces or removes all occurrences of a given word (or pattern of characters) within a character string.

- The TRANWRD function does not removed trailing blanks from *target* or *replacement*.
- If *NewVar* is not previously defined, it is given a length of 200.
- If the target string is not found in the source, then no replacement occurs.

Let's use the TRANWRD function as follows:

```
Product = Tranwrd (Product, 'Luci ', 'Lucky ');
```

First, we pass the variable to the function, in this case Product, and then tell it the target value that we want to change, which is Lucy, and finally what we are going to be replacing it with—Lucky. The function searches all observations of the product variable, looks for the term Lucy, and replaces them with Lucky.

## Creating Functions for the DATA Step

A function definition begins with the FUNCTION statement and ends with an ENDSUB statement. A SAS function is a routine that accepts arguments, performs a computation or other operation, and returns either a character or numeric value. The syntax is highly similar to the R function. The FUNCTION statement is followed by the function name and the arguments in parentheses. In addition, each function uses the RETURN statement to identify the function output.

As we learned previously, SAS has a ton of built-in functions that you can use in your DATA step. Of course, it probably doesn't have all functions that you want to use. Maybe you want to customize your own function. To do so, you will use the FUNCTION COMPILER procedure (PROC FCMP). All the functions we create here will be used inside a DATA step.

The guts of PROC FCMP are very similar to the FUNCTION function in R, as shown in Figure 3.3.

**Figure 3.3: R FUNCTION Function**

In SAS, we start with the FUNCTION statement and then specify the function name that we are going to create. Then in parentheses, we give it a list of arguments—argument 1, followed by all the other arguments—as shown in the following syntax:

**PROC FCMP OUTLIB**=*libref.data-set.package*;
    **FUNCTION** *function-name(argument-1 <$>,...,*
            *argument-n <$>) <$>; <length ;>*
            *programming-statements*;
    **RETURN**(*expression*);
    **ENDSUB**;
**QUIT**;

If the input argument is a character value, it needs a dollar sign operator. Directly after the parentheses when you have specified your input arguments, if the output value that we are creating is also a character value, we need to use the dollar sign operator again. If you are creating character data, always remember your LENGTH statement.

Then you create whatever SAS programming statements you want to offer to the function. Furthermore, PROC FCMP requires the RETURN statement, and you need to pass it the value you actually want to return. Here we can only return a single value. In later chapters, we will talk about macro programming for complete customization of SAS code where you can return as many values as you would like. And in Chapter 7 when we get into the interactive matrix language, you will learn how to create functions to return multiple matrices.

But for now, with PROC FCMP, we can only return a single value. To conclude your function, use the ENDSUB statement.

To save the functions that we create in PROC FCMP, we will use the OUTLIB option in the PROC FCMP statement. This is a three-level name that starts with the library, followed by the DATA set. We will be saving our functions in DATA sets. The third name is the actual package. We can save our functions in different packages all in a DATA set. A *package* is a collection of routines that have unique names. You can call the second and third argument of the OUTLIB option any name that you choose.

For example, maybe you have time series functions. You can save them in a specific package. Maybe you have data mining functions. You can save those in another package. And you can save all those inside a single DATA step in your library so that you can use them later in the days to come.

Let's look at an example of a PROC FCMP statement in Program 3.9. Imagine we want to switch the order of a string in a DATA set. We want to go from last, first name, to first space last name.

**Program 3.9: PROC FCMP**

```
proc fcmp outlib=work.functions.newfuncs; ❶
    function ReverseName(name $) $; ❷
    length newname $ 40; ❸
    newname=catx(' ',scan(name,2,','),scan(name,1,',')); ❹
    return(newname); ❺
    endsub; ❻
quit;
```

❶   We are saving this function in the sp4r library in the functions DATA set in the newfuncs package. The newfuncs package is a collection of routines that have unique names and are stored in the work.functions data set.

❷   Next, we have the FUNCTION statement, and we are going to call this function ReverseName. We only have one input argument, which is name, and it is a character value. The value that we are returning will also be character, so a dollar sign is needed after the parentheses.

❸   As a best practice, remember your LENGTH statement. The new value that we are creating, newname, can have up to 40 characters.

❹   Here in the function we are creating a newname variable, which is equal to the CATX function. The first argument is the delimiter, which is just a space. And then we are scanning the input argument for the second word and assuming that these words are delimited with a comma. Then we are concatenating that with the first word.

❺   Finally, you need to use a RETURN statement. We are returning the newname value.

❻   Don't forget your ENDSUB statement!


## Accessing Newly Defined Functions

Imagine you created the ReverseName function in Program 3.9, and now you want to use it, perhaps several days or weeks later. To do so, we will use the OPTIONS statement and the CMPLIB option, as shown in the following syntax:

**CMPLIB=***libref.data-set* | (*libref.data-set-1 ... libref.data-set-n*)

This is basically the same as the library function in R. The CMPLIB option is telling SAS to unpack the functions in the library in the function's DATA set. Once you unpack the functions with the OPTIONS statement, then you can use all the functions in that package.

The CMPLIB= SAS system option specifies one or more data sets that SAS searches for user-defined function entries. The default is work.functions as shown in the example function below:

```
options cmplib=work.functions;
```

The OPTIONS statement specifies or changes the value of one or more SAS system options. For example, to suppress the data that is normally written to SAS output and set a line size of 72, execute the following statement:

```
options nodate linesize=72
```

> **Tip:** Options are not saved. They must be run in each session.

### Using User-Defined Functions

Suppose that we have a data set called school and we want to add a new variable called FLName for first last name. Let's use the ReverseName function from Program 3.9 and pass it the variable name.

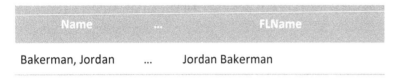

| Name | ... | FLName |
|------|-----|--------|
| Bakerman, Jordan | ... | Jordan Bakerman |

As you can see, the variable name is "Bakerman, Jordan". Program 3.10 executes the DATA step to create the new value "Jordan Bakerman" based on the ReverseName function that we created with PROC FCMP.

**Program 3.10: Using ReverseName Function**

```
options cmplib=work.functions;

data sp4r.school;
    set sp4r.school;
    FLName=ReverseName(name);
run;
```

## Subsetting Data

In this section, you will learn how to use a DATA step to subset columns, rows, and observations conditionally to a new SAS data set.

In the previous chapter, you learned how to print the unique levels of specific variables. In this section you will learn how to create a data set of those unique levels. Then in the next section, you will learn how to concatenate them together to create a data set, which is equivalent to a list in R, as shown in Figure 3.4.

**Figure 3.4: R Script**

```
 Source on Save                          Run      Source
#Identify the unique levels of the character valued variables
Make = levels(cars$Make)
Type = levels(cars$Type)
Origin = levels(cars$Origin)

#Create a list of the character valued variables
my_list = list(Make,Type,Origin)

#Create a data frame for cars from Asia
Asia = cars[cars$Origin=="Asia",]
Asia = data.frame(Asia$Name,Asia$Team,Asia$Home_Runs)

#Create a data frame for cars from Europe
Europe = cars[cars$Origin=="Europe",]
Europe = data.frame(Europe$Name,Europe$Team,Europe$Home_Runs)

#Concatenate the Boston and Montreal data frames
bos_mon = rbind(Asia,Europe)
```

Let's look at an example to learn how to subset variables in SAS. Imagine we want to pull out all the observations in the cars data set where the origin is equal to Asia, and also perhaps Europe, and then bind those rows together to create a new SAS data set.

Thus far in this book, we have specified the data set in the DATA statement and the SET statement as the same, which overwrites the existing data set with the changes. To subset a new data set, we must specify the data set we want to pull from in the SET statement and the new data set we are creating in the DATA statement, as shown in the following syntax:

**DATA** *new-data-table-name* (KEEP=*variable1 variable2 ...*)**;**
   **SET** *old-data-table-name***;**
**RUN;**

In this case, we are creating a new data set called cars2 pulling observations from cars. And as an option, we are using the KEEP= option to tell SAS that we only want to keep the variables make, msrp, and invoice. Only those three specific columns will be in the cars2 data set, as shown in Program 3.11.

**Program 3.11: Creating a New Data Set by Keeping Columns**

```
data sp4r.cars2 (keep=make msrp invoice);
    set sp4r.cars;
run;
```

Likewise, we could also create a new data set by dropping variables. In that case, we can use the DROP option, which is pretty much the same as setting the variable equal to a NULL value in your R data frame. In Program 3.12 we are creating a data set called cars2, dropping model and drive train, and keeping all other variables. The syntax is nearly identical to the KEEP= option. We just substitute DROP=.

**Program 3.12: Creating a New Data Set by Dropping Columns**

```
data sp4r.cars2 (drop=model drivetrain);
    set sp4r.cars;
run;
```

To subset by row, we can use the FIRSTOBS= and OBS= options in the SET statement as shown in the following syntax:

**DATA** *new-data-table-name***;**
   **SET** *old-data-table-name* (FIRSTOBS=# OBS=#)**;**
**RUN;**

We have seen these options previously in the PRINT procedure. In Program 3.13 we are pulling the observations 25 through 50 from the cars data set and putting them into the new cars2 data set.

**Program 3.13: Creating a New Data Set by Subsetting a Group of Observations**

```
data sp4r.cars2;
    set sp4r.cars (firstobs=25 obs=50);
run;
```

Subsetting Conditionally: WHERE Statement

We have talked about the WHERE statement during our discussion of the PRINT procedure. In that context, it was used to print observations conditionally. We can use the exact same WHERE statement and conditional expression to subset observations conditionally as shown in the following syntax:

**DATA** *new-data-table-name*;
   **SET** *old-data-table-name*;
   **WHERE** *conditional-expression*;
**RUN**;

In Program 3.14 we are creating a new data set called cars2, which is pulling all the observations from cars where mpg_city is greater than 35.

**Program 3.14: Creating a New Data Set by Subsetting Conditionally**

```
data sp4r.cars2;
    set sp4r.cars;
    where mpg_city > 35;
run;
```

The KEEP=, DROP=, FIRSTOBS=, and OBS= options can be combined with the WHERE statement to subset the data conditionally as well as according to column and row.

Subsetting by Query: PROC SQL

In the first example of PROC SQL, you learned how to print the unique levels of a specific variable. Now we will actually create a table from those unique levels. Previously we started with the SELECT UNIQUE statement, but now we will also tack on the CREATE TABLE statement as shown in the following syntax:

**PROC SQL**;
   **CREATE TABLE** *new-data-table-name* **AS**
   **SELECT UNIQUE** *variable-name* **FROM** *old-data-table-name*;
**QUIT**;

In Program 3.15 we are creating a new table in our sp4r library called origin, and then using the keyword AS. We can use the exact same syntax that we saw before to create a new table called origin and select the unique observations from origin from the cars data set. You can use as many CREATE TABLE statements as you want here to create as many new data sets as you would like as well.

**Program 3.15: Creating a New Data Set by Subsetting by Query**

```
proc sql;
    create table sp4r.origin as
    select unique origin from sp4r.cars;
quit;
```

> **Tip**: Multiple CREATE TABLE statements can be specified to create multiple data sets in a single SQL procedure.
>
> **Tip:** SELECT DISTINCT is identical to SELECT UNIQUE.

# Concatenating Data Sets

Now that we know how to subset data, what if we want to go ahead and row bind or column bind our data back together again? The following sections will explain how to reproduce the rbind() and cbind() functions in R.

## Row Bind Data Sets

To reproduce the rbind() function in R, we will use a DATA step. In the SET statement, we will specify all the data sets we want to row bind, as shown in the following syntax:

**DATA** *new-data-table-name*;
  **SET** *data-table-1 data-table-2 …* ;
**RUN**;

Let's look at an example of two data sets—employees Denmark (empsdk) and employees France (empsfr). We want to stack them on top of each other and create a new data set called employees all, as shown in Figure 3.5.

**Figure 3.5: Row Bind Data Sets**

**empsdk**

| First | Gender | Country |
|---|---|---|
| Lars | M | Denmark |
| Kari | F | Denmark |
| Jonas | M | Denmark |

**empsfr**

| First | Gender | Country |
|---|---|---|
| Pierre | M | France |
| Sophie | F | France |

**empsall**

| First | Gender | Country |
|---|---|---|
| Lars | M | Denmark |
| Kari | F | Denmark |
| Jonas | M | Denmark |
| Pierre | M | France |
| Sophie | F | France |

To do this, we will pass the employees Denmark data set and the employees France data set to a single SET statement, and it will simply stack them on top of each other as shown in Program 3.16. The important thing to remember here is the data sets have to have the exact same column names. Otherwise, you will get a block diagonal data set for empsall.

**Program 3.16: Row Bind Data Sets**

```
data empsall;
    set empsdk empsfr;
run;
```

## Column Bind Data Sets

On the other hand, if we have two separate data sets—for example, names and home—and we want to column bind them together, we will use multiple SET statements. You can think of this as creating a column of SET statements. Each SET statement should have its own data set, as shown in the following syntax:

**DATA** *new-data-table-name*;
  **SET** *data-table-1*;
  **SET** *data-table-2*;
  …
  **SET** *data-table-n*;
**RUN**;

In this case, we can set names and set home. That will column bind them to create a new SAS data set, which has the three observations, and in this case, two columns, as shown in Program 3.17 and Figure 3.6.

**Program 3.17: Column Bind Data Sets with Same Dimensions**

```
data cbind;
    set names;
    set homes;
run;
```

Figure 3.6: Column Bind Data Sets with Same Dimensions

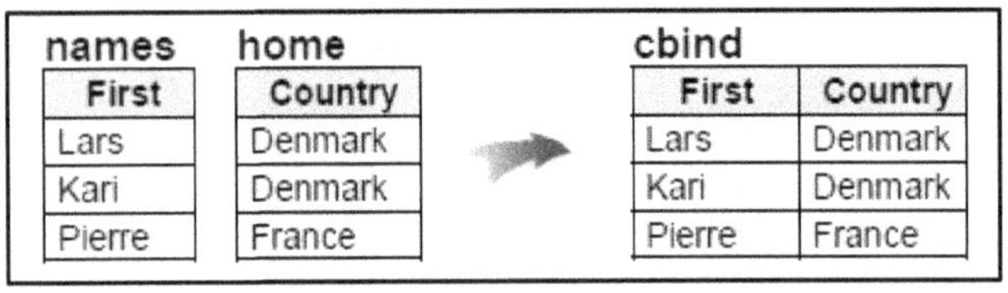

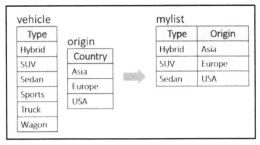

Using a SET statement to concatenate data sets of different dimensions removes observations without warning. The data set length is fixed at the length of the first data set provided in the SET statement.

To concatenate data sets of different dimensions, it is important to use the MERGE statement. For example, if we want to column bind the vehicle and origin data sets, notice that the unique levels of those two variables from the car's data set in Figure 3.6. If we use the previous syntax with multiple SET statements, SAS would actually reduce the number of observations in the final data set to only three observations as shown in Figure 3.7. SAS limits the number of observations to the smallest data set that you are merging together.

Figure 3.7: Incorrectly Column Bind Data Sets with Different Dimensions

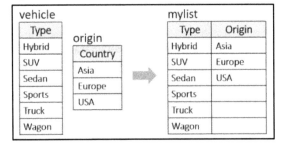

By using the MERGE statement, we are creating a list, and saving it as a SAS data set, as shown in the following syntax:

**DATA** *new-data-table-name*;
    **MERGE** *data-table-1 data-table-2 ... data-table-n*;
**RUN**;

Therefore, by using the MERGE statement, we can merge the vehicle and origin data sets together and not lose any observations as shown in Program 3.18 and Figure 3.8.

Program 3.18: Correctly Column Bind Data Sets with Different Dimensions

```
data mylist;
    merge vehicle origin;
run;
```

Figure 3.8: Correctly Column Bind Data Sets with Different Dimensions

Hopefully you can see why it's important that you use the MERGE statement for data sets with different dimensions. You could also simply use a MERGE statement every time you want to cbind if you would like.

# Match-Merging Data Sets

The MERGE statement is much more powerful than the way we used it in the previous section. Instead of just doing a straight cbind, we can actually merge according to a common variable in each data set. In the next few section, you will learn you how to do a One-to-One, One-to-Many, and Nonmatch merge, as illustrated in Figure 3.9.

**Figure 3.9: Types of Match-Merges**

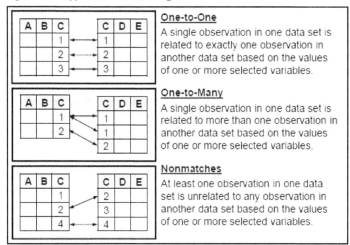

To actually do match merging, you have to first sort your data by the common variable using PROC SORT. PROC SORT is an easy procedure, which you can explore in the online documentation if you want to learn more. For now, just know that after you use the SORT procedure, you can then use your DATA step and the MERGE statement. You will list all the data sets you want to merge according to some common variable. To tell SAS what that common variable is, you will list it in the BY statement.

## One-to-One Merge

Imagine we have a data set called employees and a data set called phone, which hold the names of our employees and their phone numbers respectively, as shown in Figure 3.10. Notice that each data set has a common variable, Employee ID (EmpID). We want to merge them according to that common variable.

**Figure 3.10: One-to-One Merge Data Sets**

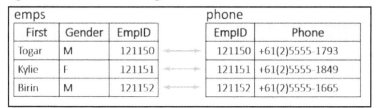

And if we did the SORT, and use the data set to do the MERGE and use the BY statement for the common variable Employee ID as shown in Program 3.19, we would get the final result in Figure 3.11. Notice that we have three observations and now only four variables.

**Program 3.19: One-to-One Merge**

```
proc sort data=emps;
   by EmpID;
run;

proc sort data=phone;
   by EmpID;
run;
```

```
data mergedemps;
    merge emps phone;
run;
```

**Figure 3.11: One-to-One Merge Results**

| First | Gender | EmpID | Phone |
|-------|--------|-------|-------|
| Togar | M | 121150 | +61(2)5555-1793 |
| Kylie | F | 121151 | +61(2)5555-1849 |
| Birin | M | 121152 | +61(2)5555-1665 |

## One-to-Many Merge

If we do a one-to-many merge, notice in Figure 3.12 that the Employee ID and the employees' data set matches to at least one Employee ID in the phone's data set.

**Figure 3.12: One-to-Many Merge Data Sets**

emps

| First | Gender | EmpID |
|-------|--------|-------|
| Togar | M | 121150 |
| Kylie | F | 121151 |
| Birin | M | 121152 |

phone

| EmpID | Type | Phone |
|-------|------|-------|
| 121150 | Home | +61(2)5555-1793 |
| 121150 | Work | +61(2)5555-1794 |
| 121151 | Home | +61(2)5555-1849 |
| 121152 | Work | +61(2)5555-1850 |
| 121152 | Home | +61(2)5555-1665 |
| 121152 | Cell | +61(2)5555-1666 |

If we do a MERGE here, the final data set would have multiple instances of the names and gender variables where it was necessary. In this instance, there are two observations for Togar because that person had two phone numbers, one for Kylie, and Birin, in this case, has three phone numbers, as shown in Figure 3.13. SAS populates the data in the new data set where necessary.

**Figure 3.13: One-to-Many Merge Results**

| First | Gender | EmpID | Type | Phone |
|-------|--------|-------|------|-------|
| Togar | M | 121150 | Home | +61(2)5555-1793 |
| Togar | M | 121150 | Work | +61(2)5555-1794 |
| Kylie | F | 121151 | Home | +61(2)5555-1849 |
| Birin | M | 121152 | Work | +61(2)5555-1850 |
| Birin | M | 121152 | Home | +61(2)5555-1665 |
| Birin | M | 121152 | Cell | +61(2)5555-1666 |

## Nonmatch Merging

Finally, to do Nonmatch merging, notice in the employees' data set in Figure 3.14 that there is one ID that does not match any ID in the phone data set. Likewise, the last observation in Employee ID does not match any Employee ID in the employees' data set.

**Figure 3.14: Nonmatch Merge Data Sets**

emps

| First | Gender | EmpID |
|-------|--------|-------|
| Togar | M | 121150 |
| Kylie | F | 121151 |
| Birin | M | 121152 |

phone

| EmpID | Phone |
|-------|-------|
| 121150 | +61(2)5555-1793 |
| 121152 | +61(2)5555-1665 |
| 121153 | +61(2)5555-1348 |

When we merge these data sets, we get exactly what we would expect. SAS just fills the data set with NULL values where necessary as shown in Figure 3.15. So Kiley does not have a phone number, and the last observation in our resulting data set has no information for first name or gender for that phone number.

**Figure 3.15: Nonmatch Merge Results**

| First | Gender | EmpID | Phone |
|-------|--------|-------|-------|
| Togar | M | 121150 | +61(2)5555-1793 |
| Kylie | F | 121151 | |
| Birin | M | 121152 | +61(2)5555-1665 |
| | | 121153 | +61(2)5555-1348 |

## Exercises

Multiple Choice

1. Choose the correct statements. (Select all that apply.)
   a. The ELSE IF and ELSE statements provide more efficient conditional processing.
   b. The DATA step uses a SET statement to add new variables to the SAS data set.
   c. You do not need to initialize the new variable.

2. Suppose you are creating a new variable called origin2 from the existing variable origin. Here you want to let origin2 be Asia if origin is 'Asia'. Otherwise, let origin2 be 'Foreign Country'. Does the DATA step below accomplish this task?

   ```
   data sp4r.cars;
       set sp4r.cars;
       length origin2 $ 25;
       if origin='Asia' then origin2='Asia';
       else origin2='Foreign Country';
   run;
   ```

   a. Yes
   b. No

3. Choose the correct statements. (Select all that apply.)
   a. DO groups enable the execution of multiple statements.
   b. Each DO group ends with an END statement.
   c. It is a best practice to use a LENGTH statement when you create character variables.

4. Which task does the DATA step below accomplish? (Choose the correct statement.)

   ```
   data sp4r.cars;
       set sp4r.cars;
       mpgvar=min(mpg_city);
   run;
   ```

   a. Return the minimum value of MPG_City.
   b. Create a new variable that is an exact duplicate of MPG_City.

5. What would the variable location be after you use the SUBSTR function?
   ```
   Location='Columbus, GA 43227';
   substr(Location,11,2)='OH';
   ```

   a. us
   b. GA
   c. OH
   d. 27

6. What is the value of the variable **location** after you use the SUBSTR function?
   ```
   data sp4r.test;
       Location='Columbus, GA 43227';
       substr(Location,11,2)='OH';
   run;
   ```

   a. Columbus, GA 43227
   b. Columbus, OH 43227

   c.   Columbus,OH 43227

   d.   an error will occur

7.   What is the value of the **newname** variable in the second observation of the **cars** data set if you run the DATA step below?

```
data sp4r.cars;
   set sp4r.cars;
   newname = upcase(catx(' ',make,scan(model,1)));
run;
```

   a.   Acura RSX

   b.   ACURA RSX

   c.   Acura RSX Type S 2dr

   d.   ACURA RSX Type S 2dr

   e.   ACURA RSX TYPE S 2DR

8.   Choose the correct statements. (Select all that apply.)

   a.   All built-in SAS functions operate the same as built-in R functions.

   b.   PROC FCMP is the counterpart to the R function function().

   c.   The CMPLIB= option in the OPTIONS statement unpacks the user-defined function.

9.   You want to use PROC FCMP to create a function that avoids division by zero. If the divisor is zero, simply return a value of zero. What is wrong with the PROC step below? Select all that apply.

```
proc fcmp outlib=sp4r.functions.newfuncs;
   function mydiv(num,den);
      if den = 0 then val = 0;
      else val = round(num/den);
   endsub;
quit;
```

   a.   It should have an ENDFUNC statement, instead of ENDSUB.

   b.   It should end with a RUN statement, instead of QUIT.

   c.   It is missing a RETURN statement to return val.

10.   Which statement and options are used to select column variables, rows, and conditional observations?

   a.   SET, DROP, KEEP

   b.   WHERE, FIRSTOBS= OBS=, SET

   c.   KEEP, FIRSTOBS= OBS=, WHERE

   d.   KEEP, WHERE, WHERE

11.   Your colleague gave you three SAS data sets and wants you to combine them into one. The data sets are unique. This means that they are of different dimensions and contain different variables. Which DATA step statements should be used to combine these data sets?

   a.   set dt1 dt2 dt3;

   b.   merge dt1 dt2 dt3;

   c.   set dt1; set dt2; set dt3;

Short Answer

1. Navigate to the SAS PROC SORT online documentation. Locate the PROC SORT statement syntax and investigate the OUT= option. What is this option used for, and what is the default behavior if it is omitted?

   Read about the caution listed in the documentation, and think of a situation in which you would need to "use care when you use PROC SORT without OUT=."

Programming Exercises

Use the **Cars** data set in the **SP4R** library to complete the exercises.

1. **Creating a New Data Set Variable**
   a. Create a new variable called **mpg_average** in the **Cars** data set. This new variable should simply be the average gas mileage between **mpg_city** and **mpg_highway**.
   b. Print the first five observations for the variables **mpg_city**, **mpg_highway**, and **mpg_average** to ensure that the new variable is created.

2. **Creating a New Data Set Variable Conditionally**
   a. Use the new variable that you created in Exercise 1. Create a new variable in the Cars data set called **mpg_quality**, which is a character variable. Set **mpg_quality** according to the following table:

   | MPG_average | MPG_quality |
   |---|---|
   | <20 | Low |
   | 20–29 | Medium |
   | >30 | High |

   b. Print observations 65 through 70 for the variables **mpg_average** and **mpg_quality** to ensure that the variable is created.

3. **Creating a New Data Set Variable Conditionally**
   a. Create a function called **tier** with a single numeric argument, which returns a character value. The function should return values according to the following table:

   | Input | output |
   |---|---|
   | <20 | Low |
   | 20–29 | Medium |
   | >30 | High |

   b. Use the function that you created to create a new variable in the Cars data set. Name the new variable **mpg_quality2** and name the argument of the function **tier** as **mpg_average**. As a result, **mpg_quality** and **mpg_quality2** are identical.
   c. Print observations 65 through 70 for the variables **mpg_average**, **mpg_quality**, and **mpg_quality2** to ensure that the variable is created.

4. **Creating a List of Unique Values**

   a. Use PROC SQL to create three new data tables. Let values of **make** be the unique levels of the **make** variable. Let the values of **type** be the unique levels of the type variable. Let the values of **origin** be the unique levels of the **origin** variable.

   b. Create a new data table called **mylist**, which combines the three data tables. Hint: This task requires you to column-bind data tables of different dimensions.

   c. Print **mylist** to ensure that the data table is created correctly.

| Obs | Make | Type | Origin |
|---|---|---|---|
| 1 | Acura | Hybrid | Asia |
| 2 | Audi | SUV | Europe |
| 3 | BMW | Sedan | USA |
| 4 | Buick | Sports | |
| 5 | Cadillac | Truck | |
| 6 | Chevrolet | Wagon | |
| 7 | Chrysler | | |
| 8 | Dodge | | |
| 9 | Ford | | |
| 10 | GMC | | |
| 11 | Honda | | |
| 12 | Hummer | | |
| 13 | Hyundai | | |
| 14 | Infiniti | | |
| 15 | Isuzu | | |
| 16 | Jaguar | | |
| 17 | Jeep | | |
| 18 | Kia | | |
| 19 | Land Rover | | |
| 20 | Lexus | | |
| 21 | Lincoln | | |
| 22 | MINI | | |
| 23 | Mazda | | |
| 24 | Mercedes-Benz | | |
| 25 | Mercury | | |
| 26 | Mitsubishi | | |
| 27 | Nissan | | |
| 28 | Oldsmobile | | |
| 29 | Pontiac | | |
| 30 | Porsche | | |
| 31 | Saab | | |
| 32 | Saturn | | |
| 33 | Scion | | |
| 34 | Subaru | | |
| 35 | Suzuki | | |
| 36 | Toyota | | |
| 37 | Volkswagen | | |
| 38 | Volvo | | |

5. **Creating and Row-Binding Data Tables**

   a. Create a new data table called **sports**, which has only three columns from the Cars data set: **make**, **type**, and **msrp**. In addition, keep only those observations where **type** is equal to *sports* and **msrp** is greater than *$100,000*.

   b. Create another data table called **suv**, which has the same three columns. In addition, keep only those observations where **type** is equal to *suv* and **msrp** is greater than *$60,000*.

   c. Create a new data table called **expensive** by row-binding **sports** and **suv**. Then print **expensive** to see the results.

| Obs | Make | Type | MSRP |
|-----|---------------|--------|-----------|
| 1 | Mercedes-Benz | Sports | $121,770 |
| 2 | Mercedes-Benz | Sports | $126,670 |
| 3 | Porsche | Sports | $192,465 |
| 4 | Land Rover | SUV | $72,250 |
| 5 | Lexus | SUV | $64,800 |
| 6 | Mercedes-Benz | SUV | $76,870 |

# Solutions

## Multiple Choice

1. a, b, and c

2. a

3. a, b, and c

4. b

5. c

6. b

7. b

8. b and c

9. c

10. c

11. b

## Short Answer

1. The OUT= option names the output data set in a PROC SORT step. Without the OUT= option, PROC SORT replaces the original data set with the sorted observations. This could result in a loss of data if the PROC SORT step includes a WHERE statement, or the FIRSTOBS or OBS option to select only a subset of the observations in the data set.

## Programming Exercises

Use the **Cars** data set in the **SP4R** library to complete the exercises.

1. **Creating a New Data Set Variable**
   a. Create a new variable called **mpg_average** in the **Cars** data set. This new variable should simply be the average gas mileage between **mpg_city** and **mpg_highway**.

   ```
   data sp4r.cars;
      set sp4r.cars;
      mpg_average = mean(mpg_city,mpg_highway);
   run;
   ```

   b. Print the first five observations for the variables **mpg_city**, **mpg_highway**, and **mpg_average** to ensure that the new variable is created.

   ```
   proc print data=sp4r.cars (obs=5);
      var mpg_city mpg_highway mpg_average;
   run;
   ```

   | Obs | MPG_City | MPG_<br>Highway | mpg_<br>average |
   |-----|----------|---------|---------|
   | 1 | 17 | 23 | 20.0 |
   | 2 | 24 | 31 | 27.5 |
   | 3 | 22 | 29 | 25.5 |
   | 4 | 20 | 28 | 24.0 |
   | 5 | 18 | 24 | 21.0 |

2.   **Creating a New Data Set Variable Conditionally**

a.   Use the new variable that you created in Exercise 1. Create a new variable in the Cars data set called **mpg_quality**, which is a character variable. Set **mpg_quality** according to the following table:

| MPG_average | MPG_quality |
|-------------|-------------|
| <20 | Low |
| 20–29 | Medium |
| >30 | High |

```
data sp4r.cars;
    length mpg_quality $ 6;
    set sp4r.cars;
    if mpg_average < 20 then mpg_quality='Low';
    else if mpg_average < 30 then mpg_quality='Medium';
    else mpg_quality='High';
run;
```

b.   Print observations 65 through 70 for the variables **mpg_average** and **mpg_quality** to ensure that the variable is created.

```
proc print data=sp4r.cars (firstobs=65 obs=70);
    var mpg_average mpg_quality;
run;
```

| Obs | mpg_ average | mpg_ quality |
|-----|------|------|
| 65 | 16.0 | Low |
| 66 | 18.5 | Low |
| 67 | 20.5 | Medium |
| 68 | 31.0 | High |
| 69 | 31.0 | High |
| 70 | 31.5 | High |

3.   **Creating a New Data Set Variable Conditionally**

a.   Create a function called **tier** with a single numeric argument, which returns a character value. The function should return values according to the following table:

| Input | output |
|-------|--------|
| <20 | Low |
| 20–29 | Medium |
| >30 | High |

```
proc fcmp outlib=work.functions.newfuncs;
    function tier(val) $;
        length newval $ 6;
        if val < 20 then newval = 'Low';
        else if val <30 then newval='Medium';
            else newval='High';
        return(newval);
      endsub;
quit;
```

b.  Use the function that you created to create a new variable in the Cars data set. Name the new variable **mpg_quality2** and name the argument of the function **tier** as **mpg_average**. As a result, **mpg_quality** and **mpg_quality2** are identical.

```
options cmplib=work.functions;
data sp4r.cars;
    set sp4r.cars;
    mpg_quality2=tier(mpg_average);
run;
```

c.  Print observations 65 through 70 for the variables **mpg_average**, **mpg_quality**, and **mpg_quality2** to ensure that the variable is created.

```
proc print data=sp4r.cars (firstobs=65 obs=70);
    var mpg_average mpg_quality mpg_quality2;
run;
```

| Obs | mpg_ average | mpg_ quality | mpg_ quality2 |
|-----|--------------|--------------|---------------|
| 65  | 16.0         | Low          | Low           |
| 66  | 18.5         | Low          | Low           |
| 67  | 20.5         | Medium       | Medium        |
| 68  | 31.0         | High         | High          |
| 69  | 31.0         | High         | High          |
| 70  | 31.5         | High         | High          |

4.  **Creating a List of Unique Values**

a.  Use PROC SQL to create three new data tables. Let values of **make** be the unique levels of the **make** variable. Let the values of **type** be the unique levels of the type variable. Let the values of **origin** be the unique levels of the **origin** variable.

```
proc sql;
    create table make as select unique make from sp4r.cars;
    create table type as select unique type from sp4r.cars;
    create table origin as select unique origin from
        sp4r.cars;
quit;
```

b.  Create a new data table called **mylist**, which combines the three data tables. Hint: This task requires you to column-bind data tables of different dimensions.

```
data sp4r.mylist;
    merge make type origin;
run;
```

c.  Print **mylist** to ensure that the data table is created correctly.

```
proc print data=sp4r.mylist;
run;
```

```
Obs     Make            Type      Origin

 1      Acura           Hybrid    Asia
 2      Audi            SUV       Europe
 3      BMW             Sedan     USA
 4      Buick           Sports
 5      Cadillac        Truck
 6      Chevrolet       Wagon
 7      Chrysler
 8      Dodge
 9      Ford
10      GMC
11      Honda
12      Hummer
13      Hyundai
14      Infiniti
15      Isuzu
16      Jaguar
17      Jeep
18      Kia
19      Land Rover
20      Lexus
21      Lincoln
22      MINI
23      Mazda
24      Mercedes-Benz
25      Mercury
26      Mitsubishi
27      Nissan
28      Oldsmobile
29      Pontiac
30      Porsche
31      Saab
32      Saturn
33      Scion
34      Subaru
35      Suzuki
36      Toyota
37      Volkswagen
38      Volvo
```

5. **Creating and Row-Binding Data Tables**
   a. Create a new data table called **sports**, which has only three columns from the Cars data set: **make**, **type**, and **msrp**. In addition, keep only those observations where **type** is equal to *sports* and **msrp** is greater than *$100,000*.

   ```
   data sp4r.sports(keep= make type msrp);
       set sp4r.cars;
       where type='Sports' and msrp>100000;
   run;
   ```

   b. Create another data table called **suv**, which has the same three columns. In addition, keep only those observations where **type** is equal to *suv* and **msrp** is greater than *$60,000*.

   ```
   data sp4r.suv(keep= make type msrp);
       set sp4r.cars;
       where type='SUV' and msrp>60000;
   run;
   ```

   c. Create a new data table called **expensive** by row-binding **sports** and **suv**. Then print **expensive** to see the results.

   ```
   data sp4r.expensive;
       set sp4r.sports sp4r.suv;
   run;

   proc print data= sp4r.expensive;
   run;
   ```

   ```
   Obs     Make              Type      MSRP

    1      Mercedes-Benz     Sports    $121,770
    2      Mercedes-Benz     Sports    $126,670
    3      Porsche           Sports    $192,465
    4      Land Rover        SUV        $72,250
    5      Lexus             SUV        $64,800
    6      Mercedes-Benz     SUV        $76,870
   ```

# Chapter 4: Random Number Generation and Plotting

## Introduction

Creating statistical graphics is vital to understanding and presenting your data. In this chapter, you will learn how to create a variety of both single-cell and multi-cell plots. We will create everything from histograms to scatter plots inside a single procedure and enhance the presentation of the plot with an assortment of statements and options. Before we create statistical graphics, we will first learn how to simulate new SAS data sets from probability distributions so that we can generate data from a desired model. We will then create and use these random data sets to practice building a variety of plots.

## DO Loop and Random Number Generation

In this section, you will learn how to simulate observations from random distributions like the normal, chi-square, gamma, and Weibull distributions and save those observations in a new SAS data table. We want to be able to set a seed so that we can duplicate our results. We want to create random data sets from our R functions in R, rnorm, rbinom, and so on. We also want to be able to add variables to an existing data frame as shown in Figure 4.1. Maybe we also want to use the REP function to create a classification variable. And finally, we want to use the other probability functions, like dnorm pnorm, and qnorm.

**Figure 4.1: R Script**

```
                                                                    Run      Source
#Set a seed for random number generation
set.seed(123)

#Create a data set of random numbers
n=10
random - cbind(rnorm(n,20,5),rbinom(n,1,.25),runif(n,0,10),rexp(n,1.5))

#Add a random vector to the data set
random = cbind(random, rgeom(n,.1))

#Group random numbers
group - rep(1:5,each-3)
n-length(group)
random - cbind(group,1:n,rpois(n,25),rbeta(n,.5,.5))

#Find Density, CDF, and Quantile of distribution
q - seq(-3,3,by-.5)
d = dnorm(q,0,1)
p - pnorm(q,0,1)
random - cbind(q,d,p,qnorm(p,0,1))
```

## DO Loop

To duplicate this script in SAS, we need to use the DO loop. The DO loop is the key to creating a new data table. The number of loop iterations defines the table's row dimension and the number of variables defines the column dimension. The DO loop is used inside a DATA step to create new data tables or iterate through rows of an existing data table.

We can create a sequence, maybe 1 to 10, 2 to 20 by 2. Or we can go in the reverse order. Maybe we want to create repetitive values. For example, maybe we want to add a column of 1s to a data table, which will represent an intercept if we are simulating a linear regression model. We want to be able to create groups such as, for example, a classification variable if we are simulating ANOVA data. In particular, we are going to focus on generating random numbers and creating a new SAS data set.

The DO loop is equivalent to the seq() function in R. You can also think of it as a FOR loop. In SAS, we start with a DO statement and specify an index variable as shown in the following syntax:

**DO** *index-variable=start* **TO** *stop* <**BY** *increment*>;
**END**;

Let's look at a simple example with an index variable, i, in the following DO loop:

```
do i=1 to 5;
end;
```

We will set i equal to a starting value of 1. Use the keyword TO to give it a stopping value—in this case, 5. So we are going from i equals 1 to 5. It acts as a sequence. Always end your DO loop with the END statement.

Below are a two more examples of DO loops. In the first loop, we add in the BY increment option. In this loop, we are going from i equals 2 to 10 by 2. We can also reverse direction, as shown in the second loop where i equals 10 to 2 by negative 2.

```
do i=2 to 10 by 2;
end;
```

```
do i=10 to 2 by -2;
end;
```

You can create a new SAS data set using the DATA step and a DO loop, as shown in the following syntax:

**DATA** *data-table-name-new*;
  **DO** *index-variable=start* **TO** *stop* <**BY** *increment*>;
    *iterated-SAS-statements*;
  **OUTPUT**;
  **END**;
**RUN**;

> **Tip:** Omitting the BY statement causes the DO loop to iterate by 1.

The number of DO loop iterations determines the number of observations that are written to the data table when you use the OUTPUT statement. In Program 4.1, we are going from i equals 2 to 10 and giving an increment of 2. In order to actually output all iteration values to the data set loop, we need to use the OUTPUT statement. Otherwise, SAS would only write the last value of the loop. There would only be one observation if we forget the OUTPUT statement. You need to be explicit and tell SAS to write all iteration values to the data set. And again, remember to end the DO loop with an END statement.

**Program 4.1: Create New Data Set**

```
data loop;
    do i=2 to 10 by 2;
        x = i+1;
        rep = 1;
        output;
    end;
run;
```

Inside the loop in Program 4.1, we have created a new variable, x. We are saying that x is equal to the index variable, i, plus 1. We are also creating a new variable rep, which just equals 1 in every instance of the iteration. In Output 4.1, which shows the PROC PRINT of the loop data set, the index variable, i, is 2 to 10, x is 3 to 11, and rep is just 1, which would most likely represent an intercept in the linear model.

**Output 4.1: Results of Program 4.1**

| Obs | i | x | rep |
|---|---|---|---|
| 1 | 2 | 3 | 1 |
| 2 | 4 | 5 | 1 |
| 3 | 6 | 7 | 1 |
| 4 | 8 | 9 | 1 |
| 5 | 10 | 11 | 1 |

If you don't want to keep your index variable in your data set, you have two options. You can specify the KEEP= or DROP= options in the DATA statement. In Program 4.2a, we use the KEEP= option in the DATA statement to keep only the variables x and rep.

**Program 4.2a: KEEP= Option**

```
data loop (keep=x rep);
    do i=2 to 10 by 2;
        x = i+1;
        rep = 1;
        output;
    end;
run;
```

Likewise, you can tell SAS to drop that index variable, i, using the DROP= option as shown in Program 4.2b.

**Program 4.2b: DROP= Option**

```
data loop (drop=i);
    do i=2 to 10 by 2;
        x = i+1;
        rep = 1;
        output;
    end;
run;
```

Both DATA steps produce the same data table, as shown in Output 4.2. Use the KEEP or DROP statement depending on the ease of variable specification.

**Output 4.2: Results of Program 4.2a or 4.2b**

| Obs | x | rep |
|-----|-----|-----|
| 1 | 3 | 1 |
| 2 | 5 | 1 |
| 3 | 7 | 1 |
| 4 | 9 | 1 |
| 5 | 11 | 1 |

Nested DO Loop

A nested DO loop is similar to the REP function in R show in Figure 4.2. It allows us to repeat values. It's also similar to a nested FOR loop. A nested DO loop can be used to replicate the predecessor DO loop variables and to create groups.

**Figure 4.2: R REP Function**

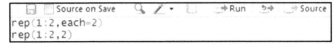

```
rep(1:2,each=2)
rep(1:2,2)
```

Program 4.3 shows a nested DO loop going from i equals 1 to 2. Immediately following it, we have another DO loop, j equals 1 to 2. Of course, remember your OUTPUT statement to write all your values to the data table.

**Program 4.3: Nested DO Loop**

```
do i=1 to 2;
    do j=1 to 2;
        output;
    end;
end;
```

Notice that in Output 4.3, in iteration i, we start with a value of 1 and iterate through j, 1 and 2. And then moving to a value of 2 for i, we iterate again through j, 1 and 2. This is exactly the same as the FOR loop in R.

**Output 4.3: Results of Program 4.3**

| Obs | i | j |
|-----|-----|-----|
| 1 | 1 | 1 |
| 2 | 1 | 2 |
| 3 | 2 | 1 |
| 4 | 2 | 2 |

There is an alternative way to accomplish the nested DO loop. Applying a DO loop to an existing data table has the same effect as a nested DO loop. You can just use multiple DO loops in sequential DATA steps. In Program 4.4, we are creating the data set doloop. Here we are going from i equals 1 to 2, and writing both values to the data table.

**Program 4.4: Create Data Set**

```
data doloop;
    do i=1 to 2;
        output;
    end;
run;
```

In Program 4.5, we then apply another DO loop to an existing SAS data set-- in this case, the doloop data set created in Program 4.4. The DO loop will iterate through all observations in that data set. It's going to iterate through values of 1 and 2 for the index variable i.

**Program 4.5: Apply Do Loop to Existing Data Set**

```
data doloop;
    set doloop;
    do j=1 to 2;
        output;
    end;
run;
```

Output 4.5 shows that we get the same data set as before in Output 4.3 when we used the nested DO loop.

**Output 4.5: Results of Program 4.5**

| Obs | i | j |
|-----|---|---|
| 1 | 1 | 1 |
| 2 | 1 | 2 |
| 3 | 2 | 1 |
| 4 | 2 | 2 |

Why is this important? Well, perhaps you want to go ahead and add a sequence to an existing data set but you don't want to use another DO loop on that existing data set. For example, if you have a data set with 1,000 observations and you want to create a sequence from 1 to 1,000 and add it into that data set. You do not want to use a DO loop. Why? It will simply create a data set with 1,000 by 1,000 observations, or simply 1,000,000 observations.

So how can we add in a sequence to an existing SAS data set? This will be important when plot data so that we can give the plots an X-axis value. To add in a sequence, we will use a SUM statement, which is discussed in the next section.

SUM Statement

The SUM statement creates a new variable. Use a SUM statement to add a sequence to

- an existing data table
- a nested DO loop

The variable is automatically initialized to zero and its value is retained from one iteration of the DATA step to the next. On each iteration, the new variable is incremented by the sequence value. The SUM statement can be useful when you add a sequence to a data table. Use the following syntax to add a SUM statement:

*new-variable-name* + *sequence-value*;

In Program 4.6, we are calling our SUM statement seq. And that will be the variable name in the data set. We give it the sequence value of 1. So seq plus 1. When we start the DATA step, it initializes to 0. And on the first iteration, the value is going to be 0 plus 1. We use the OUTPUT statement so the value is written to the data table. And on the next iteration, the seq value is 2, 3, and so on. Basically, we use a SUM statement to add a sequence to an existing SAS data set.

**Program 4.6: SUM Statement**

```
data doloop;
    do i=1 to 2;
        do j=1 to 2;
            seq + 1;
            output;
        end;
    end;
run;
```

**Output 4.6: Results of Program 4.6**

| Obs | i | j | seq |
|-----|---|---|-----|
| 1 | 1 | 1 | 1 |
| 2 | 1 | 2 | 2 |
| 3 | 2 | 1 | 3 |
| 4 | 2 | 2 | 4 |

## Random Number Generation

Why is the DO loop so important? It specifies how many random numbers to generate. The DO loop is used to simultaneously create a data table and generate random numbers to let us create new SAS data sets. Now we can use the DO loop to assist in creating random number distribution data tables.

### RAND Function

We will use the RAND function inside the DO loop—which is going to be used, of course, inside the DATA step—to create new SAS data sets.

To sample from random probability distributions, we use the RAND function. The RAND function is very similar to the R functions in R. Table 4.1 shows a sample list comparing the syntax between R and SAS.

**Table 4.1: Comparing R and SAS**

| R | SAS |
|---|-----|
| rbinom(n,size,p) | RAND('Binomial',p,n) |
| rexp(n,rate) | RAND('Exponential') |
| rnorm(n,mean,sd) | RAND('Normal',mean,sd) |
| rpois(n,mean) | RAND('Poisson',mean) |
| runif(n,min,max) | RAND('Uniform') |

The first argument in the RAND function is just the name of the distribution. And you do have to put it in quotation marks. The next set of arguments is the parameters for that specific distribution, as shown in the following syntax:

RAND('*distribution*',*param-1*,*param-2*,…);

Make sure you check the online documentation page for the RAND function so that you know what probability distributions you can simulate. You also need to know the order of the parameters.

You may have noticed in Table 4.1 that not all probability distributions are the same in R as they are in SAS. So, for example, the Exponential distribution actually does not have a mean or rate parameter. You have to multiply the distribution by its mean to do the equivalent. The Uniform distribution in SAS only simulates values between 0 and 1. So, for example, if you wanted a distribution between 0 and 10, you would simply multiply all simulated values by 10.

In Program 4.7, we are going to create a new data set called random.

**Program 4.7: RAND Function in DO Loop**

```
data random (drop=i); ❶
    call streaminit(123); ❷
    do i=1 to 3;
        x = rand('Normal',10,2); ❸
        output; ❹
```

```
    end;
run;
```

❶ Here we drop the index variable, i.

❷ We use the STREAMINIT subroutine to set a seed to 123.

❸ Then we use a DO loop where i equals 1 to 3, creating a new variable, x, which is equal to the RAND function. It's going to be normally distributed data set with a mean of 10 and a standard deviation of 2.

❹ Of course, don't forget the OUTPUT statement to write all values to the data table.

Notice in Program 4.7 that we don't have to specify a number of the values to simulate directly in the RAND function. That is taken care of inside the DO loop. Because we are entering from 1 to 3—that is, entering three total values—the RAND function is going to create three simulated values.

If you want to add a column of random numbers to an existing data set, do not use the DO loop. Simply use your SET statement and create a new variable as shown in Program 4.8. In this case, we are creating the variable x, which is equal to the RAND function again.

**Program 4.8: RAND Function Without DO Loop**

```
data sp4r.cars;
    call streaminit(123);
    set sp4r.cars;
    x = rand('Normal',10,2);
run;
```

Again, in Program 4.8, you don't need to specify a number to simulate. It's going to simulate the total number of observations in the existing data set. If the cars data set has 428 observations, the RAND function will generate 428 observations as well.

## Other Probability Functions

Let's look at just a few other functions. When we generate random numbers, we can use the PDF, CDF, and QUANTILE functions. They operate the exact same way in SAS as they do in R.

Let's look at an example of how to duplicate the dnorm, pnorm, and qnorm functions with the PDF, CDF, and QUANTILE functions in Table 4.2.

**Table 4.2: PDF, CDF, and QUANTILE Functions with R Counterparts**

| R | SAS |
| --- | --- |
| dnorm(q,mean, sd) | PDF('Normal',q,mean,sd) |
| pnorm(q,mean,sd) | CDF('Normal',q,mean,sd) |
| qnorm(p,mean,sd) | QUANTILE('Normal',p,mean,sd) |

As you can see in Table 4.2, we specify the distribution name. In this case, it is Normal. Then we give it either the quantile for the PDF and CDF function or the cumulative distribution for the QUANTILE function. The final two arguments are the parameters for the distribution. In this case, they are mean and standard deviation.

> **TIP:** You can also use these functions in a DATA _NULL_ step to print the results of these SAS functions to the log.

## Single-Cell Plotting with PROC SGPLOT

Now that we know how to create our own random data sets, let's plot those data sets and practice the plotting capabilities in SAS. In this section, we will learn how to reproduce the base R plotting capabilities shown in Figure 4.3 including a bar plot, box plot, histogram with some overlaid normal and kernel density estimates, simple linear regression plot with the line of best fit, confidence limits, and prediction limits.

**Figure 4.3: R Script and Plots**

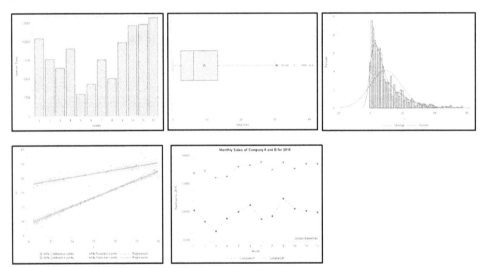

```
                                              Source on Save        Run        Source
#Create histogram with density estimate
n=300; vec = rexp(n,1/10); s = rep(1:3,each=100)
hist(vec, 50,freq=F)
lines(density(vec),col="red")

#Create boxplot
boxplot(vec~s,horizontal=T)

#Create bar chart
n=12; vec = rnorm(12,10000,5000)
barplot(vec)

#Create scatter plot
x = 1:30; y1 = 10+x+rnorm(30); y2 = 35+x/2+rnorm(30)
plot(y1~x,ylim=c(10,50)); abline(lm(y1~x))
points(y2~x); abline(lm(y2~x))

#Enhance the Plot
x = 1:12
revenue = rnorm(12,10000,1000)
revenue_2 = rnorm(12,13000,500)
plot(revenue~x,type="b",col="blue",ylim=c(8000,14000),
    main="Monthly Sale of Company A and B for 2015",
    xlab="Month",ylab="Revenue for 2015",pch=16,lty=2)
lines(revenue_2~x,type="b",col="red",pch=16,lty=2)
text(10,8000,"Jordan B")
abline(h=11000,col="grey"); abline(v=6.5,col="grey")
legend(2,9500,c("A","B"),col=c("blue","red"),lty=c(2,2))
```

At the end of this section, you will learn how to touch up your plots and make a nice visual presentation by adding a title, a different legend, and even your name so that you can take credit for your plot. You can also change the pattern of the lines, the symbols for the points, change the x and y labels, and so on.

## PROC SGPLOT Syntax

All of the plotting capabilities in R can be accomplished in SAS by the SGPLOT procedure. SGPLOT stands for statistical graphics plot. We can create single-cell plots just like the plot function in R. We can also overlay plots on a single set of axes. If we want to overlay two scatterplots on a single plot, we can do that using PROC SGPLOT. And finally, we will enhance the presentation of the plot with different options and statements in PROC SGPLOT.

Table 4.3 lists a few plots that you can create in PROC SGPLOT organized into four categories. To view the rest of the plots the SGPLOT procedure can produce, go to the SAS Documentation where you can also view options and other statements.

**Table 4.3: SGPLOT Procedure Plot Types**

| Type | Plots | PLOT Statement |
|---|---|---|
| Basic | scatter, series, step, needle, vector, bubble, and band | SCATTER, SERIES, STEP, NEEDLE, VECTOR, BUBBLE, BAND |
| Fit and Confidence | regression, loess, penalized B-spline curves, ellipses | REG, LOESS, PBSPLINE, ELLIPSE |
| Distribution | box plot, histogram, normal/kernel density | HBOX, VBOX, HISTOGRAM, DENSITY |
| Categorical | bar chart, line chart, and dot plots | HBAR, VBAR, HLINE, VLINE, DOT |

The SGPLOT procedure statements conform to different syntaxes depending on the plot type. For the Basic and Fit-and-Confidence plot types, specify the PLOT statement followed by the X-axis variable and the Y-axis variable as shown below:

**PLOTNAME** X=*x-variable* Y=*y-variable* </ OPTIONS>;

For example, if you want to create a scatterplot, you would simply use the SCATTER statement in the SGPLOT procedure. Likewise, if you wanted to create a series plot, you would just use the SERIES statement. Under the PROC SGPLOT umbrella, you are just changing out your statements to use a different plot.

For the Distribution and Categorical plot types, specify the PLOT statement followed by the response variable as shown in the following syntax:

**PLOTNAME** *response-or-category-variable* </ OPTIONS>;

For example, if you want a bivariate plot, scatter, series, regression, or loess, you use the PLOT statement that is appropriate. Then you use the x equal to and y equal to options to specify your X-axis and Y-axis variables. And you can specify options right in the statement after the forward slash.

This syntax is very consistent going forward in SAS. We will see the forward slash to denote options both in PROC SGPLOT and lots of inferential procedures in Chapter 6. Be sure to look at the online documentation page to see all the possible options for the procedure. You can do a lot of different fancy things with different options, depending on the plot.

There are two basic plot types that have slightly different syntax. The band plot, of course, is bivariate, but it has some different options. You do need the X-axis variable, but you also need the lower and upper option to specify where exactly you are going to be shading in a region. So what region are you shading in between a lower bound and upper bound for your band plot? For a Band plot, specify the X-axis variable followed by the lower and upper region to be filled, as shown below:

**BAND** X=*x-variable* LOWER=*lower-bound* UPPER=*upper-bound*;

And finally, for the bubble plot, you do specify the x- and y-axis variables because it is a scatterplot. You also use the size option to specify how big you want each bubble to be, which is based on another variable in your existing SAS data set. For a bubble plot, specify the X-axis variable, y-axis variable, and a numeric variable to alter the size of the scatter plot points with the following syntax:

**BUBBLE** X=x-variable Y=y-variable SIZE=size-variable;

## Scatterplot Example

Imagine we have a data set called sales, which holds the revenue for each of the 12 months this past year. We want to create a scatterplot with a SCATTER statement and let the X-axis variable be month, and Y-axis variable be revenue. Using the syntax in Program 4.9 will produce the exact same plot as using the plot function in R, as shown in Output 4.9.

**Program 4.9: PROC SGPLOT with a Single SCATTER Statement**

```
proc sgplot data=sales;
    scatter x=month y=revenue;
run;
```

**Output 4.9: Results of Program 4.9**

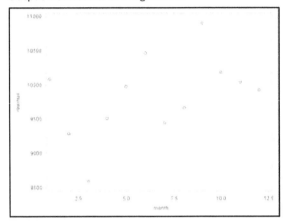

In R, you generally create a plot and then iteratively add options to the plot. For example, you would create a scatterplot and then you could use the points or lines function to overlay either another scatterplot or a series plot on top of it. In SAS, we do everything in one PROC step. We don't iteratively add graphics to an existing plot.

For example, if you wanted to create multiple scatterplots in a single window, which basically reproduces the points function in R, we would just use multiple SCATTER statements. In Program 4.10, we have the same x variable, but now we have two separate y variables—y equal to revenue and y equal to revenue 2.

**Program 4.10: PROC SGPLOT with a Multiple SCATTER Statements**

```
proc sgplot data=sales;
    scatter x=month y=revenue;
    scatter x=month y=revenue_2;
run;
```

**Output 4.10: Results of Program 4.10**

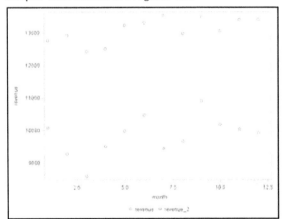

As you can see in Output 4.10, it plots the first revenue in blue and the second revenue in red. Again, this would replicate the points function in R.

If we were simply just to switch out the SCATTER statements with SERIES statements as shown in Program 4.11, it would reproduce the lines function in R. The SGPLOT procedure automatically populates a legend when multiple SCATTER or SERIES statements are provided.

**Program 4.11: PROC SGPLOT with a Multiple SERIES Statements**

```
proc sgplot data=sales;
    series x=month y=revenue;
    series x=month y=revenue_2;
run;
```

**Output 4.11: Results of Program 4.11**

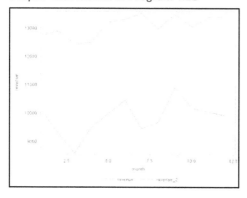

Generally, you can use whatever PLOT statements you want. However, there does have to be some structure. For example, you cannot use the SCATTER statement and also the BOX PLOT statement. Those two plots are not capable of being in the same window.

## Alternative Overlay Approach

Alternative overlay approaches depend on the structure of the data table. Imagine we have a data set called sales, but this time, we have a variable called company, which is a classification variable. A value of 1 indicates company1. A value 2 indicates company2. Month and revenue are stacked as shown in Figure 4.4.

**Figure 4.4: Sales Data Set**

| Obs | company | month | revenue |
|-----|---------|-------|---------|
| 1   | 1       | 1     | 10083.94 |
| 2   | 1       | 2     | 9287.52 |
| ... |         |       |         |
| 12  | 1       | 12    | 9923.39 |
| 13  | 2       | 1     | 12761.45 |
| 14  | 2       | 2     | 12905.25 |
| ... |         |       |         |
| 24  | 2       | 12    | 13403.48 |

How can we reproduce the points function in this instance? We can one SCATTER statement, as shown in Program 4.12. As an option after the forward slash, we will use the group equal to option and give it the classification variable. This tells SAS to divide up the job. Now we are plotting revenue and revenue2 separately on the same plot, which looks the same as Output 4.10.

**Program 4.12: PROC SGPLOT with GROUP= Option**

```
proc sgplot data=sales;
    scatter x=month y=revenue / group=company;
run;
```

If the response variables are stacked, another approach is to use the BY statement and plot the two companies separately. In Program 4.13, we pass the BY statement the classification variable, and SAS prints the scatterplot for company1 and then company2 separately as shown in Output 4.13.

**Program 4.13: PROC SGPLOT with BY statement**

```
proc sgplot data=sales;
    scatter x=month y=revenue
    by company;
run;
```

**Output 4.13: Results of Program 4.13**

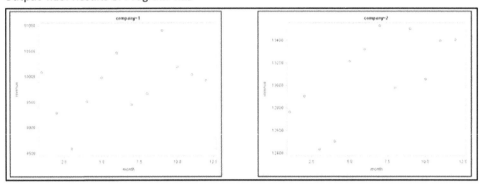

To review, the BY statement produces a plot for each category of the specified variable. Use the GROUP= option to overlay and the BY statement to output multiple plots. We will see the BY statement again going forward in this course. It's very consistent in most procedures. We will see it in Chapter 7 when we start using simulations for some more efficient SAS programming.

## Multi-Cell Plotting with Procedures and Statements

In this section, you will learn how to create multi-cell plots. You will learn how to create a window and fill the window with different types of plots like a histogram, density estimate, and a box plot. We will also explore how to create a scatter-plot matrix, and finally, create a panel of plots based on some classification variable.

In R, we would use the PAIRS function to create a scatter-plot matrix, and we would also be comfortable using the PAR MFROW option to create a window and fill that window with different types of plots. The R script that we will attempt to duplicate in this section is shown in Figure 4.5.

**Figure 4.5: R Script**

```
 Source on Save    Run    Source
#Create a scatter plot matrix
n - 1000
x = rexp(n)
y = rnorm(n,3,1)
z = rchisq(n,10)
pairs(~x+y+z)

#Create side by side histograms
n-1000
fem = rnorm(n,66,2)
mal = rnorm(n,72,2)
par(mfrow=c(1,2))
hist(fem,50,main="Histogram of Female Heights")
hist(mal,50,main="Histogram of Female Heights")

#Create a window with multiple plots
n-1000
fem - rnorm(n,66,2)
par(mfrow=c(1,3))
hist(fem,50,main="Histogram of Female Heights")
plot(density(fem),main="Density Estimate of Female Heights")
boxplot(fem,main="Boxplot of Female Heights")
```

## PROC SGSCATTER

First, let's talk about the SGSCATTER procedure, which creates a paneled graph of scatter plots depending on the PLOT statement that you use. There are three different PLOT statements that we can use with PROC SGSCATTER:

- the MATRIX statement creates a scatter-plot matrix to duplicate the pairs() function in R
- the PLOT statement creates a paneled graph that contains multiple independent scatter plots
- the COMPARE statement creates a comparative panel of scatter plots based on shared axes

### MATRIX Statement

First, in PROC SGSCATTER, if we use the MATRIX statement, we simply specify all the variables we want to include in the scatter-plot matrix as shown in the following syntax:

**MATRIX** *variable-1 variable-2 … </ options>*;

In Program 4.14, we are creating a scatter-plot matrix of mpg_city, weight, and length. Options in the MATRIX statement enable both histograms and density estimates to be plotted on the diagonal of the scatter plot matrix.

**Program 4.14: PROC SGSCATTER with MATRIX Statement**
```
proc sgscatter data=sp4r.cars;
    matrix mpg_city weight length;
run;
```

**Output 4.14: Results of Program 4.14**

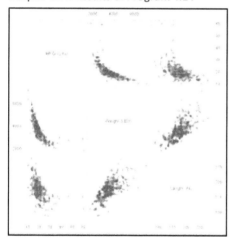

### PLOT Statement

Next, using the PLOT statement, we can create multi-cell scatter plots. In the PLOT statement, we cross whatever variables we want to create a scatter plot for in our data set, as shown in the following syntax:

**PLOT** *variable-i \* variable-j … </ options>*;

In Program 4.15, we first create a scatter plot of mpg_city by weight, then create a scatter plot of mpg_city by length, and finally, weight by length. As an option, you can use the ROWS= and COLUMNS= to specify the structure of the graphic.

**Program 4.15: PROC SGSCATTER with PLOT Statement**
```
proc sgscatter data=sp4r.cars;
    plot mpg_city*weight mpg_city*length
    weight*length / columns=3;
run;
```

In Output 4.15, you can see that we have one row and three columns for these three scatter plots.

**Output 4.15: Results of Program 4.15**

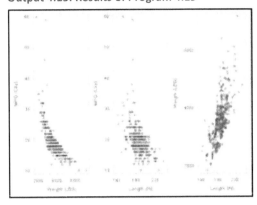

COMPARE Statement

Finally, we can use the COMPARE statement to create a comparative panel of scatter plots according to some shared axes. We will always use the Y= and X= option, and in parentheses, give it the y or x variables as shown in the following syntax:

**COMPARE** X=(*variable-i...*) Y=(*variable-j...*)... *</ options>*;

The dimension of the graph is determined by the number of variables in the Y= and X= statements. So in Program 4.16, for the Y-axis variable, we are specifying mpg_city, which is going to be the shared axes variable, and the X-axis variables will be weight and length. This means we are going to create scatter plots of mpg_city by weight and mpg_city by length.

**Program 4.16: PROC SGSCATTER with COMPARE Statement**

```
proc sgscatter data=sp4r.cars;
    compare y=(mpg_city) x=(weight length);
run;
```

As you can see in the plot in Output 4.16, there is no Y-axis variable for the second plot because it is a shared axis.

**Output 4.16: Results of Program 4.16**

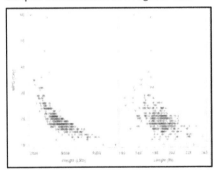

## ODS LAYOUT Statements

### ODS LAYOUT START

To combine plots of different types, use the ODS LAYOUT statement. To reproduce the par(mfrow=c(,)) function in R, we will use the ODS LAYOUT START statement with the following syntax:

**ODS LAYOUT START** ROWS= COLUMNS=
           &lt;WIDTH= HEIGHT= ROW_HEIGHT=
           COLUMN_HEIGHT=ROW_GUTTER=
           COLUMN_GUTTER=*options*&gt;;

**ODS LAYOUT END;**

In the same way that we pass the number of rows and columns to the PAR MFROW function in R as arguments, we use the ROWS= and COLUMNS= options to specify the structure of the new window. Once we specify the structure, we can then fill the window with whatever plots we want.

There are lots of different options for the ODS LAYOUT statement. For example, use ROW_HEIGHT, COLUMN_HEIGHT to specify the heights of the plots that you are creating. Use ROW_GUTTER and COLUMN_GUTTER to reduce or increase the space between consecutive plots, and so on.

Once you are done filling the window, you should use the ODS LAYOUT END statement. That lets SAS go back to the default plotting requirements, which is similar to turning off the PAR function in R.

### ODS REGION

Once we use the ODS LAYOUT START statement, we will then use the ODS REGION statement to specify the location of each plot by using the following syntax:

**ODS REGION** ROW= COLUMN=;

So, for example, in Program 4.17, in row one, column three, we are going to fit the following plot: a horizontal box plot for mpg_city.

**Program 4.17: ODS REGION Statement**
```
ods region row=1 column=3;
    proc sgplot data=sp4r.cars;
    hbox mpg_city;
run;
```

ODS REGION tells SAS exactly where to put the plot in your window, and if you don't use the ODS REGION, it will just specify them consecutively. It will start in the top left corner, filling all the way to the bottom right corner of your window.

But of course, in this example, we only have one row and three columns, so it would start by filling the leftmost column and ending with the rightmost column.

## PROC SGPANEL

The SGPANEL procedure is used to create a panel of plots according to a classification variable. The SGPANEL procedure combines plots of the same type only. The panel automatically generates a title for each plot according to the classification variable.

Imagine we have a histogram for the mpg_city variable in the cars data set that is for all the observations in my data set, but perhaps we want to split it up and create histograms for each level of the origin variable.

If we want to create a histogram for ORIGIN= Asia, Europe, and USA, we can use the SGPANEL procedure with the following options:

**PANELBY** *classification-variable*;

**PLOTNAME** *response-or-category-variable </ options>*;

PROC SGPANEL is followed by the PANELBY statement, which enables the user to specify a classification variable. The panel creates the same plot type for each classification and response. All the plot types from the "Single-Cell Plotting" section can be used with PROC SGPANEL.

Program 4.18 shows how to create a histogram for the levels of origin separately. Here, all the observations for Asia, Europe, and USA are plotted separately.

**Program 4.18: PROC SGPANEL**

```
proc sgpanel data=sp4r.cars;
    panelby origin / columns=3;
    histogram mpg_city;
run;
```

**Output 4.18: Results of Program 4.18**

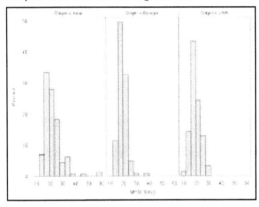

You can specify multiple classification variables in your PANELBY statement, and SAS will simply cross all classification levels of each variable as shown in Program 4.19. Again, use your ROWS and COLUMNS options to specify structure for your window.

**Program 4.19: PROC SGPANEL with Multiple Classification Variables**

```
proc sgpanel data=sp4r.lesscars;
    panelby origin type / rows=1 columns=4;
    reg x=weight y=mpg_city;
run;
```

**Output 4.19: Results of Program 4.19**

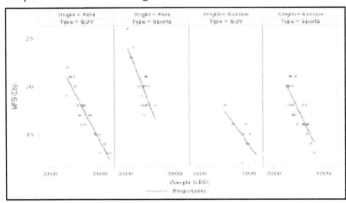

Program 4.19 uses the REG statement to add in a line of best fit for simple linear regression data: X-axis variable (weight), and Y-axis variable (mpg_city). Notice that the title of each plot specifies the classification level for each variable, origin, and type.

# Exercises

1. Does the following DO loop create a data table with a sequence from 50 to 100 by 5 with the variable name myloop?

```
data doloop;
   do myloop=50 to 100 by 5;
   end;
run;
```

   a. Yes
   b. No

2. What is the dimension of the data set created below?

```
 data random;
    do i=1 to 3;
       do j=1 to 2;
          do k=1 to 2;
             output;
          end;
       end;
    end;
 run;
```

   a. 12x12
   b. 6x3
   c. 8x3
   d. 12x3

3. Do the SAS functions rand('Beta',5,7) and CDF('Beta',.3,5,7) reproduce the R functions rbeta(1,5,7) and pbeta(.3,5,7)?
   a. Yes
   b. No

4. Navigate to the SGPLOT procedure HELP documentation and examine the plotting statements. Which statement was used to create the following plot?

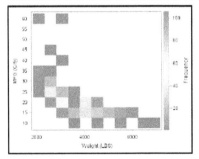

   a. HEATMAP
   b. POLYGON
   c. BUBBLE
   d. BLOCK

5. Which SGPLOT procedure statement was used to create the following plot?

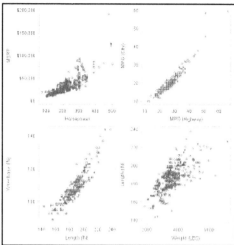

    a.    MATRIX

    b.    PLOT

    c.    COMPARE

## Programming Exercises

1. **Using the DO loop and Creating Random Data Sets**

    a.    Navigate to the **SAS RAND function** page and choose a few functions to practice generating random numbers. Create a data table with at least two variables of random numbers and at least 10 observations. Be sure to use a random seed of your choice.

         http://support.sas.com/documentation/cdl/en/lefunctionsref/67960/HTML/default/viewer.htm#p0fpeei0opypg8n1b06qe4r040lv.htm

    b.    Create a new data table with the same random variables that you specified from the previous step. Create a variable called **Class** that groups the first five observations into class 1 and the second five into class 2. Drop the nested DO loop index variable from the data table and add a sequence from 1 to 10. Print the data upon completion.

    c.    Run the SAS code below. What do you notice?

```
data test;
    do i=1 to 2;
        output;
    end;
run;

proc print data=test;
run;

data test;
    set test;
    do j=1 to 5;
        output;
    end;
run;

proc print data=test;
run;
```

2. **Exploring PDF, CDF, and Quantiles Variables**

    a.    Use the DO loop to create quantiles from 0 to 10 by 1.

    b.    Identify the density and the cumulative density of a binomial distribution with parameters 0.8 and 10 by creating variables **PDF** and **CDF**.

    c.    Use the **CDF** variable to create the variable **Quantile**, which mirrors the DO loop values.

    d.    Print the data upon completion.

3. **Plotting Chi-Square Random Numbers**

   a. Create a data table with 1000 random deviates from a chi-square distribution with 20 degrees of freedom and a seed of 123.

   b. Use PROC SGPLOT to plot a histogram of the data.

      1) Alter the appearance of the plot by setting the BINWIDTH= option to 1.

      2) Add both a normal and kernel density estimate.

      3) Add the title 'My Random Chi-Square Distribution'.

      4) Add the X-axis title 'Random Chi-Square Deviates'.

      5) Use X-axis limits of 5 and 40.

      6) Request the frequency instead of the percent by providing the option SCALE=COUNT in the HISTOGRAM statement.

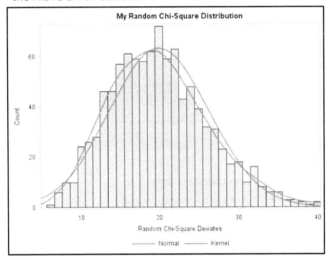

4. **Plotting Simple Linear Regression Data**

   a. Create a data table with $Y = \beta_0 + \beta_1 X + \varepsilon$ where $X$ ranges from 1 to 30, $\beta_0 = 25$, $\beta_1 = 1$, and $\varepsilon \sim N(\mu = 0, \sigma = 5)$. Keep only the variables $X$ and $Y$.

   b. Use PROC SGPLOT and the REG statement to plot the line of best fit for the data. Create a plot of the data. Use both the SCATTER and REG statement to plot the points and a line of best fit.

      a. Enhance the plot by coloring the points blue and using the symbol STARFILLED

      b. Color the regression line red and use the pattern DOT.

      c. Add a title of your choosing to the X axis, Y axis, and the main title.

      d. Use the X-axis limits from 0 to 31, and the Y-axis limits from 15 to 65.

      e. Name the legend 'Scatter' and 'Line of Best Fit' for both plot types.

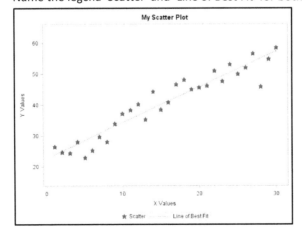

c. Alter the previous plot by changing the SCATTER statement to NEEDLE and the REG statement to PBSPLINE. (This demonstrates the ease in which plot types can be altered.)

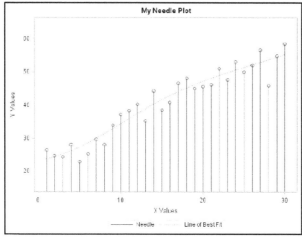

5. **Creating a Bubble Plot**

   a. Create a data table with two groups of 20 and the random seed 123. Create two random variables. Let the first be exponential and the second be binomial with parameters 0.5 and 5.

   b. Use the BUBBLE statement to create a bubble plot. Set the SIZE= to the binomial random variable. Also, specify the GROUP= option based on the two separate groups. Finally, provide the plot with titles for the X axis, Y axis, and main title.

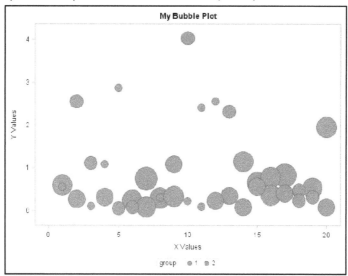

6. **Using PROC SGSCATTER**

   a. Create a data table with 300 observations and a seed of 123.

      i. Let X be the deviates from the standard normal distribution.

      ii. Produce a variable Y1, which is X plus standard normal deviates.

      iii. Produce another variable such that Y2 is 5*X plus standard normal deviates.

b. Use PROC SGSCATTER to create a scatter plot matrix of X, Y1, and Y2. Include histograms and kernel density estimates on the diagonal. (Hint: Look up the DIAGONAL= option in the MATRIX statement of the SGSCATTER procedure.)

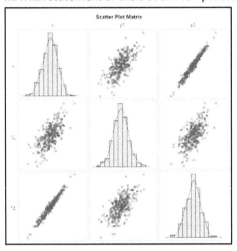

c. Use PROC SGSCATTER to create side-by-side scatter plots of Y1 by X and Y2 by X with the PLOT statement. Add the regression line to both plots with the REG option.

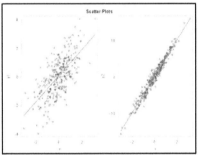

d. Use PROC SGSCATTER and the COMPARE statement to create the same scatter plot with shared axes.

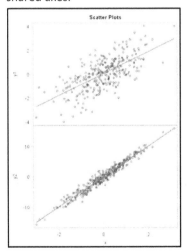

7. **Using PROC SGPANEL**

   a. Instead of creating Y1 and Y2 as separate variables from the previous exercise, stack the variables in a single column denoted Y using a nested DO loop.

      i. Create a categorical variable called Year with groups 1 and 2.

      ii. Generate 300 observations for each group with a random seed of 123.

      iii. Let X be the deviates from a standard normal distribution.

    iv.    Use IF-THEN/ELSE syntax to let Y be X plus standard normal deviates if Year is 1 and let Y be 5*X plus standard normal deviates otherwise.

b.    Use PROC SGPANEL to create a regression panel by year.

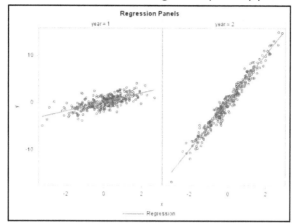

## Solutions

### Multiple Choice

1. b – In order to save all values of each iteration, you must use the OUTPUT statement.
2. d – The number of iterations for nested DO loops is the product of the number of iterations for each index (3x2x2=12). In addition, we did not drop any of the three indices, so the data set dimension is 12x3.
3. a – The RAND and CDF function in SAS are equivalent to the r and p probability functions in R. The only difference is in SAS, we do not specify the number of iterations in the function when simulating new data.
4. a – The heat map here color codes the cells in the bivariate plot according to the frequency of observations in each cell.
5. b – This plot was created using the PLOT statement because we have a window of four independent scatter plots. The plot was not created using the MATRIX statement because the diagonal element would not be scatterplots and it was not created using the COMPARE statement because there are no shared axes.

### Programming Exercises

1. **Using the DO loop and Creating Random Data Sets**
    a. Navigate to the **SAS RAND function** page and choose a few functions to practice generating random numbers. Create a data table with at least two variables of random numbers and at least 10 observations. Be sure to use a random seed of your choice.

```
data sp4r.random;
    call streaminit(123);
    do i=1 to 10;
        rt = rand('T',5);
        rf = rand('F',3,4);
        ru = int(rand('Uniform')*10);
        output;
    end;
run;

proc print data=sp4r.random;
run;
```

| Obs | i | rt | rf | ru |
|---|---|---|---|---|
| 1 | 1 | 0.15554 | 0.57611 | 3 |
| 2 | 2 | -0.71020 | 0.15053 | 2 |
| 3 | 3 | -0.02583 | 0.04516 | 9 |
| 4 | 4 | 0.73364 | 0.25261 | 7 |
| 5 | 5 | 0.18336 | 0.88293 | 4 |
| 6 | 6 | 0.13730 | 1.50425 | 9 |
| 7 | 7 | 0.90893 | 2.18254 | 9 |
| 8 | 8 | 0.04611 | 0.10342 | 8 |
| 9 | 9 | 2.41523 | 0.55436 | 5 |
| 10 | 10 | 0.20044 | 1.59396 | 1 |

    b. Create a new data table with the same random variables that you specified from the previous step. Create a variable called **Class** that groups the first five observations into class 1 and the second five into class 2. Drop the nested DO loop index variable from the data table and add a sequence from 1 to 10. Print the data upon completion.

```
data sp4r.random (drop=j);
    call streaminit(123);
    do class=1 to 2;
        do j=1 to 5;
            sequence + 1;
            rt = rand('T',5);
            rf = rand('F',3,4);
            ru = int(rand('Uniform')*10);
```

```
                output;
            end;
        end;
    run;

    proc print data=sp4r.random;
    run;
```

| Obs | class | sequence | rt | rf | ru |
|-----|-------|----------|------|------|-----|
| 1 | 1 | 1 | 0.15554 | 0.57611 | 3 |
| 2 | 1 | 2 | -0.71020 | 0.15053 | 2 |
| 3 | 1 | 3 | -0.02583 | 0.04516 | 9 |
| 4 | 1 | 4 | 0.73364 | 0.25261 | 7 |
| 5 | 1 | 5 | 0.18336 | 0.88293 | 4 |
| 6 | 2 | 6 | 0.13730 | 1.50425 | 9 |
| 7 | 2 | 7 | 0.90693 | 2.18254 | 9 |
| 8 | 2 | 8 | 0.04611 | 0.10342 | 8 |
| 9 | 2 | 9 | 2.41523 | 0.55436 | 5 |
| 10 | 2 | 10 | 0.20044 | 1.59396 | 1 |

c.  Run the SAS code below. What do you notice?

```
data test;
    do i=1 to 2;
        output;
    end;
run;

proc print data=test;
run;

data test;
    set test;
    do j=1 to 5;
        output;
    end;
run;

proc print data=test;
run;
```

**The loop iterates through each observation in the data table.**

2. **Exploring PDF, CDF, and Quantiles Variables**
    a.  Use the DO loop to create quantiles from 0 to 10 by 1.
    b.  Identify the density and the cumulative density of a binomial distribution with parameters 0.8 and 10 by creating variables **PDF** and **CDF**.
    c.  Use the **CDF** variable to create the variable **Quantile**, which mirrors the DO loop values.
    d.  Print the data upon completion.

```
data sp4r.random;
    do q=0 to 10 by 1;
        pdf = pdf('Binomial',q,.8,10);
        cdf = cdf('Binomial',q,.8,10);
        quantile = quantile('Binomial',cdf,.8,10);
        output;
    end;
run;

proc print data=sp4r.random;
run;
```

| Obs | q | pdf | cdf | quantile |
|---|---|---|---|---|
| 1 | 0 | 0.00000 | 0.00000 | 0 |
| 2 | 1 | 0.00000 | 0.00000 | 1 |
| 3 | 2 | 0.00007 | 0.00008 | 2 |
| 4 | 3 | 0.00079 | 0.00086 | 3 |
| 5 | 4 | 0.00551 | 0.00637 | 4 |
| 6 | 5 | 0.02642 | 0.03279 | 5 |
| 7 | 6 | 0.08808 | 0.12087 | 6 |
| 8 | 7 | 0.20133 | 0.32220 | 7 |
| 9 | 8 | 0.30199 | 0.62419 | 8 |
| 10 | 9 | 0.26844 | 0.89263 | 9 |
| 11 | 10 | 0.10737 | 1.00000 | 10 |

3. **Plotting Chi-Square Random Numbers**

   a.   Create a data table with 1000 random deviates from a chi-square distribution with 20 degrees of freedom and a seed of 123.

```
data sp4r.hist;
    call streaminit(123);
    do i=1 to 1000;
        rchisq = rand('chisquare',20);
        output;
    end;
run;
```

   b.   Use PROC SGPLOT to plot a histogram of the data.

   1)   Alter the appearance of the plot by setting the BINWIDTH= option to 1.

   2)   Add both a normal and kernel density estimate.

   3)   Add the title 'My Random Chi-Square Distribution'.

   4)   Add the X-axis title 'Random Chi-Square Deviates'.

   5)   Use X-axis limits of 5 and 40.

   6)   Request the frequency instead of the percent by providing the option SCALE=COUNT in the HISTOGRAM statement.

```
proc sgplot data=sp4r.hist;
    histogram rchisq / binwidth=1 scale=count;
    density rchisq / type=normal;
    density rchisq / type=kernel;
    title 'My Random Chi-Square Distribution';
    xaxis label='Random Chi-Square Deviates' min=5 max=40;
run;
```

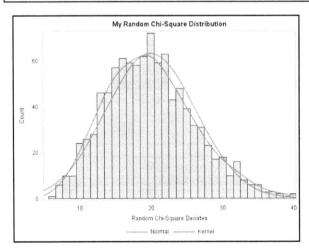

4. **Plotting Simple Linear Regression Data**

   a. Create a data table with $Y = \beta_0 + \beta_1 X + \varepsilon$ where $X$ ranges from 1 to 30, $\beta_0 = 25$, $\beta_1 = 1$, and $\varepsilon \sim N(\mu = 0, \sigma = 5)$. Keep only the variables $X$ and $Y$.

```
data sp4r.simple_lin (keep=x y);
    call streaminit(123);
    do x=1 to 30;
        beta01 = 25;
        beta11 = 1;
        y = beta01 + beta11*x + rand('Normal',0,5);
        output;
    end;
run;
```

   b. Use PROC SGPLOT and the REG statement to plot the line of best fit for the data. Create a plot of the data. Use both the SCATTER and REG statement to plot the points and a line of best fit.

      a. Enhance the plot by coloring the points blue and using the symbol STARFILLED

      b. Color the regression line red and use the pattern DOT.

      c. Add a title of your choosing to the X axis, Y axis, and the main title.

      d. Use the X-axis limits from 0 to 31, and the Y-axis limits from 15 to 65.

      e. Name the legend 'Scatter' and 'Line of Best Fit' for both plot types.

```
proc sgplot data=sp4r.simple_lin;
    scatter x=x y=y / legendlabel='Scatter' name='Scatter'
      markerattrs=(color=blue symbol=starfilled);
    reg x=x y=y / legendlabel='Line of Best Fit' name='Line'
      lineattrs=(color=red pattern=dot);

    title 'My Scatter Plot';
    xaxis label='X Values' min=0 max=31;
    yaxis label='Y Values' min=15 max=65;
    keylegend 'Scatter' 'Line';
run;
```

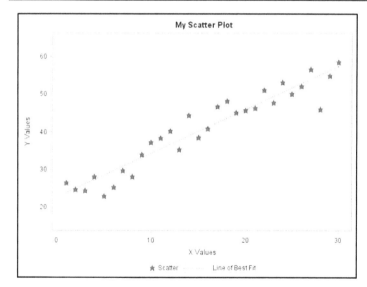

c. Alter the previous plot by changing the SCATTER statement to NEEDLE and the REG statement to PBSPLINE. (This demonstrates the ease in which plot types can be altered.)

```
proc sgplot data=sp4r.simple_lin;
    needle x=x y=y / legendlabel='Needle' name='Needle'
markerattrs=(color=blue symbol=starfilled);
    pbspline x=x y=y / legendlabel='Line of Best Fit'
        name='Line'
        lineattrs=(color=red pattern=dot);

    title 'My Needle Plot';
    xaxis label='X Values' min=0 max=31;
    yaxis label='Y Values' min=15 max=65;
    keylegend 'Needle' 'Line';
run;
```

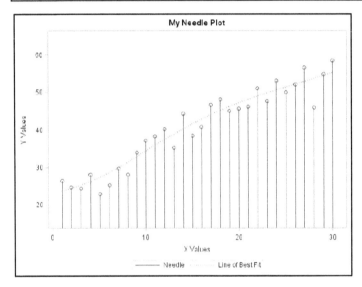

5. **Creating a Bubble Plot**

a. Create a data table with two groups of 20 and the random seed 123. Create two random variables. Let the first be exponential and the second be binomial with parameters 0.5 and 5.

```
data sp4r.bubble;
    call streaminit(123);
    do group=1 to 2;
        do x=1 to 20;
            y = rand('Exponential');
            z = rand('binomial',.5,5);
            output;
        end;
    end;
run;
```

b. Use the BUBBLE statement to create a bubble plot. Set the SIZE= to the binomial random variable. Also, specify the GROUP= option based on the two separate groups. Finally, provide the plot with titles for the X axis, Y axis, and main title.

```
proc sgplot data=sp4r.bubble;
    bubble x=x y=y size=z / group=group;

    title 'My Bubble Plot';
    xaxis label='X Values';
    yaxis label='Y Values';
run;
```

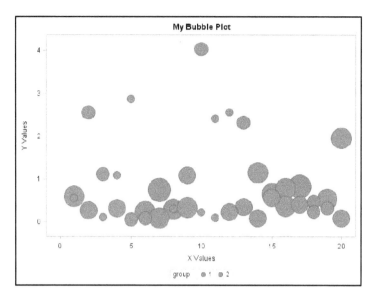

6. **Using PROC SGSCATTER**

   a. Create a data table with 300 observations and a seed of 123.

      i. Let X be the deviates from the standard normal distribution.

      ii. Produce a variable Y1, which is X plus standard normal deviates.

      iii. Produce another variable such that Y2 is 5*X plus standard normal deviates.

```
data sp4r.random;
    call streaminit(123);
    do i=1 to 300;
        x = rand('Normal');
        y1 = x + rand('Normal');
        y2 = 5*x + rand('Normal');
        output;
    end;
run;
```

   b. Use PROC SGSCATTER to create a scatter plot matrix of X, Y1, and Y2. Include histograms and kernel density estimates on the diagonal. (Hint: Look up the DIAGONAL= option in the MATRIX statement of the SGSCATTER procedure.)

```
proc sgscatter data=sp4r.random;
    matrix x y1 y2 / diagonal=(histogram kernel);
    title 'Scatter Plot Matrix';
run;
title;
```

   Selected PROC SGSCATTER statement and option:

   MATRIX specifies the variables used to create a scatter plot matrix. Use the DIAGONAL= option to include a histogram, density estimates, or both as the diagonal elements of the scatter plot matrix.

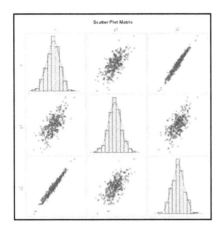

c.  Use PROC SGSCATTER to create side-by-side scatter plots of Y1 by X and Y2 by X with the PLOT statement. Add the regression line to both plots with the REG option.

```
proc sgscatter data=sp4r.random;
    plot (y1 y2) * x / reg;
    title 'Scatter Plots';
run;
title;
```

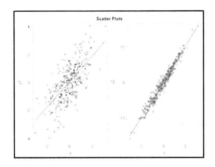

d.  Use PROC SGSCATTER and the COMPARE statement to create the same scatter plot with shared axes.

```
proc sgscatter;
    compare y=(y1 y2) x=x / reg;
    title 'Scatter Plots';
run;
title;
```

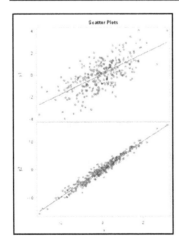

7. **Using PROC SGPANEL**
    a. Instead of creating Y1 and Y2 as separate variables from the previous exercise, stack the variables in a single column denoted Y using a nested DO loop.
        i. Create a categorical variable called Year with groups 1 and 2.
        ii. Generate 300 observations for each group with a random seed of 123.
        iii. Let X be the deviates from a standard normal distribution.
        iv. Use IF-THEN/ELSE syntax to let Y be X plus standard normal deviates if Year is 1 and let Y be 5*X plus standard normal deviates otherwise.

```
data sp4r.random;
    call streaminit(123);
    do year=1 to 2;
        do j=1 to 300;
            x = rand('Normal');
            if year=1 then y = x + rand('Normal');
            if year=2 then y = 5*x + rand('Normal');
            output;
        end;
    end;
run;
```

    b. Use PROC SGPANEL to create a regression panel by year.

```
proc sgpanel data=sp4r.random;
    panelby year;
    reg x=x y=y;
    title 'Regression Panels';
run;
title;
```

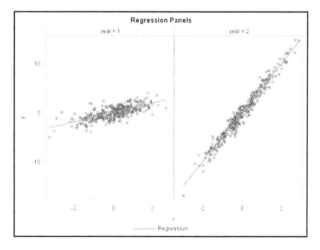

# Chapter 5: Descriptive Procedures, Output Delivery System, and Macros

## Introduction

You might find this chapter to be more challenging than the previous ones. We will start by talking about the four go-to procedures for generating summary statistics: PROC CORR, PROC FREQ, PROC MEANS, and PROC UNIVARIATE.

Next, we will talk about the Output Delivery System (ODS), which from an R user's perspective can be used to customize and save the generated output. Remember, SAS does not save output in objects, so to parallelize the approach of pulling fields from an object, we can use ODS statements.

The second half of this chapter examines macro variables and macro programs. By now you have noticed that the scope of variables is specific to the data set that you are working with. What if we want to create a global variable that can be passed to any procedure or DATA step? We can use macro variables.

Finally, we will learn how to create macros programs, which you can think of simply as an R function. This will enable you to customize and automate the generation of SAS code. We will write macro programs that generate and execute DATA and PROC steps automatically based on the parameters that we pass in the macro call.

## Summary Statistics Procedures

This section introduces four different procedures to analyze variables and generate summary statistics. We will reproduce the COR and COV functions in R as shown in Figure 5.1, as well as the TABLE function for frequency tables of classification variables. We will also generate the qqnorm plot, which is not in PROC SGPLOT. And we will compute summary statistics like mean, median, mode, range, and so on. These will be applied to the entire column or variable of your data set.

**Figure 5.1: R Script**

```
          Source on Save    Q  /  ▾                        → Run    2+    → Source
#Compute correlation and covariance matrices
cor(cbind(cars$Horsepower,cars$Weight,cars$Length))
cov(cbind(cars$Horsepower,cars$Weight,cars$Length))

#Create frequency tables
table(cars$Origin)
table(cars$Type)
#Create contingency tables
table(cars$Origin,cars$Type)

#Create QQ-plot
qqnorm(cars$Hits)

#Compute summary statistics
mean(cars$mpg_city)
median(cars$mpg_city)
mode(cars$mpg_city)
range(cars$mpg_city)
var(cars$mpg_city)
sd(cars$mpg_city)
sum(cars$mpg_city)
min(cars$mpg_city)
max(cars$mpg_city)
quantile(cars$mpg_city,c(.01,.05,.1,.25,.5,.75,.05,.9,.99))
```

Remember in Chapter 3 that we used functions in the DATA step, and they were only applied across rows. In this section, for these procedures, they will operate on the entire variable.

### PROC CORR

PROC CORR does exactly what you expect: it makes a correlation matrix. In the VAR statement of PROC CORR, we list all the variables we want added into the correlation matrix, as shown in the following syntax:

**PROC CORR DATA=**=*SAS-data-set <options>*;
   **VAR** *variable-1 … variable-n*;
**RUN;**

> **Tip:** If no VAR statement is included, all numeric variables in the data set are included.

For example, in Program 5.1 using the cars data set, we list the variables horsepower, weight, and length in the VAR statement.

**Program 5.1: PROC CORR**

```
proc corr data=sp4r.cars;
    var horsepower weight length;
run;
```

**Output 5.1: Results of Program 5.1**

| Simple Statistics | | | | | | |
|---|---|---|---|---|---|---|
| Variable | N | Mean | Std Dev | Sum | Minimum | Maximum |
| Horsepower | 428 | 215.88551 | 71.83603 | 92399 | 73.00000 | 500.00000 |
| Weight | 428 | 3578 | 758.98321 | 1531364 | 1850 | 7190 |
| Length | 428 | 186.36215 | 14.35799 | 79763 | 143.00000 | 238.00000 |

| Pearson Correlation Coefficients, N = 428 Prob > \|r\| under H0: Rho=0 | | | |
|---|---|---|---|
| | Horsepower | Weight | Length |
| Horsepower | 1.00000 | 0.63080 < .0001 | 0.38155 < .0001 |
| Weight | 0.63080 < .0001 | 1.00000 | 0.69002 < .0001 |
| Length | 0.38155 < .0001 | 0.69002 < .0001 | 1.00000 |

Notice that the second table in Output 5.1 is the Correlation Matrix. There are two values in each cell. The first value is the estimated correlation, and the second is the hypothesis test *p*-value, testing the population correlation coefficient. For example, the correlation coefficient between Horsepower and Weight is 0.63. And the *p*-value is less than 0.001, meaning it is highly significant.

Also, by default in the output, we get the Simple Statistics table. This shows the number of observations (N), the Mean, Standard Deviation, Sum, Minimum, and Maximum for our three variables as well.

Program 5.2 and Output 5.2 show that if you tack on the COV option in the PROC CORR statement, in addition to the previous tables, we get the Covariance Matrix, which is the same as the COV function in R.

**Program 5.2: PROC CORR with COV Option**

```
proc corr data=sp4r.cars cov;
    var horsepower weight length;
run;
```

**Output 5.2: Partial Results of Program 5.2**

| Covariance Matrix, DF = 427 | | | |
|---|---|---|---|
| | Horsepower | Weight | Length |
| Horsepower | 5160.4154 | 34392.4654 | 393.5427 |
| Weight | 34392.4654 | 576055.5201 | 7519.4830 |
| Length | 393.5427 | 7519.4830 | 206.1519 |

As you can see, there are lots and lots of different options that you can specify in these Summary Statistics procedures.

## PROC FREQ

Next, when working with categorical data, we can use PROC FREQ to create frequency tables. Instead of the VAR statement as we did with PROC CORR, we use the TABLES statement as shown in the following syntax:

**PROC FREQ DATA=***SAS-data-set* *<options>*;
    **TABLES** *variable-1 ... variable-n* / *<options>*;
**RUN;**

> **Tip:** If the TABLES statement is omitted, a one-way frequency table is produced for every variable in the data set. This is seldom preferred. Therefore, simply specify all the one-way frequency tables that you want to generate in the TABLE statement.

In Program 5.3, we will generate two separate tables for Origin and Type shown in Output 4.3.

**Program 5.3: PROC FREQ**

```
proc freq data=sp4r.cars;
    tables origin type;
run;
```

**Output 5.3: Results of Program 5.3**

| Origin | Frequency | Percent | Cumulative Frequency | Cumulative Percent |
|--------|-----------|---------|----------------------|--------------------|
| Asia   | 158       | 36.92   | 158                  | 36.92              |
| Europe | 123       | 28.74   | 281                  | 65.65              |
| USA    | 147       | 34.35   | 428                  | 100.00             |

| Type   | Frequency | Percent | Cumulative Frequency | Cumulative Percent |
|--------|-----------|---------|----------------------|--------------------|
| Hybrid | 3         | 0.70    | 3                    | 0.70               |
| SUV    | 60        | 14.02   | 63                   | 14.72              |
| Sedan  | 262       | 61.21   | 325                  | 75.93              |
| Sports | 49        | 11.45   | 374                  | 87.38              |
| Truck  | 24        | 5.61    | 398                  | 92.99              |
| Wagon  | 30        | 7.01    | 428                  | 100.00             |

As you can see in Output 5.3, we get the Frequency for each level of each variable. By default, we also get the percentage of observations in that level, as well as the Cumulative Frequency and Cumulative Percent.

## Cross Tabulation

If you want to do a cross tabulation, simply cross your variables in the TABLE statement with the star operator. Program 5.4 and Output 5.4 shows how to cross Origin and Type.

**Program 5.4: PROC FREQ Cross Tabulation**

```
proc freq data=sp4r.cars;
    tables origin*type;
run;
```

**Output 5.4: Results of Program 2.4**

| Frequency Percent Row Pct Col Pct | Table of Origin by Type | | | | | | |
|---|---|---|---|---|---|---|---|
| | | | Type | | | | |
| Origin | Hybrid | SUV | Sedan | Sports | Truck | Wagon | Total |
| Asia | 3 | 25 | 94 | 17 | 8 | 11 | 158 |
|  | 0.70 | 5.84 | 21.96 | 3.97 | 1.87 | 2.57 | 36.92 |
|  | 1.90 | 15.82 | 59.49 | 10.76 | 5.06 | 6.96 | |
|  | 100.00 | 41.67 | 35.88 | 34.69 | 33.33 | 36.67 | |
| Europe | 0 | 10 | 78 | 23 | 0 | 12 | 123 |
|  | 0.00 | 2.34 | 18.22 | 5.37 | 0.00 | 2.80 | 28.74 |
|  | 0.00 | 8.13 | 63.41 | 18.70 | 0.00 | 9.76 | |
|  | 0.00 | 16.67 | 29.77 | 46.94 | 0.00 | 40.00 | |
| USA | 0 | 25 | 90 | 9 | 16 | 7 | 147 |
|  | 0.00 | 5.84 | 21.03 | 2.10 | 3.74 | 1.64 | 34.35 |
|  | 0.00 | 17.01 | 61.22 | 6.12 | 10.88 | 4.76 | |
|  | 0.00 | 41.67 | 34.35 | 18.37 | 66.67 | 23.33 | |
| Total | 3 | 60 | 262 | 49 | 24 | 30 | 428 |
|  | 0.70 | 14.02 | 61.21 | 11.45 | 5.61 | 7.01 | 100.00 |

In each cell of Output 5.4, we have the Frequency, Percent, Row Percent, and Col Percent, just like we saw before. For example, all three vehicles that were hybrid vehicles came from Asia. And that corresponded to only 0.7% of our data. And on the bottom, and far right of the table, we get the totals.

## Options

If you want to reproduce your tables exactly like you would see them in R, you can use options in the TABLES statement to suppress the display of selected default statistics. Specifically, we can suppress the rows, columns, the percentage, and the frequency if we want, as shown in Table 5.1.

**Table 5.1: Options to Suppress Statistics**

| Option | Description |
| --- | --- |
| NOROW | Suppresses the display of the row percentage. |
| NOCOL | Suppresses the display of the column percentage. |
| NOPERCENT | Suppresses the percentage display. |
| NOFREQ | Suppresses the frequency display |

It's unlikely that you would want to use the NOFREQ option, but you can if you would like. In Program 5.5, we are reproducing the table() function exactly as you would see it in R. In the TABLE statement, we are crossing Origin and Type. After the forward slash, specify norow, nocol, and nopercent so that all we have in each cell are the Frequencies.

**Program 5.5: PROC FREQ with Suppress Statistics Options**

```
proc freq data=sp4r.cars;
tables origin*type / norow nocol nopercent;
run;
```

**Output 5.5: Results of Program 5.5**

| Frequency | Table of Origin by Type | | | | | | |
| --- | --- | --- | --- | --- | --- | --- | --- |
| | | | Type | | | | |
| Origin | Hybrid | SUV | Sedan | Sports | Truck | Wagon | Total |
| Asia | 3 | 25 | 94 | 17 | 8 | 11 | 158 |
| Europe | 0 | 10 | 78 | 23 | 0 | 12 | 123 |
| USA | 0 | 25 | 90 | 9 | 16 | 7 | 147 |
| Total | 3 | 60 | 262 | 49 | 24 | 30 | 428 |

Previously with PROC SQL, you saw how to print the unique levels of a variable. But perhaps there are hundreds, maybe even thousands, of levels in a specific variable. What if we just want to print the number of levels in each variable? In the PROC FREQ statement, use the nlevels option as shown in Program 5.6.

**Program 5.6: PROC FREQ with NLEVELS Option**

```
proc freq data=sp4r.cars nlevels;
tables origin*type /
norow nocol nopercent noprint;
run;
```

**Output 5.6: Results of Program 5.6**

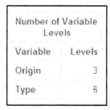

| Number of Variable Levels | |
| --- | --- |
| Variable | Levels |
| Origin | 3 |
| Type | 6 |

Output 5.6 shows the number of variable levels. For Origin, of course, there's only three levels, and for Type, there's only six levels. If you don't want to print the original frequency tables, you can use the NOPRINT option in the TABLE statement.

## PROC MEANS

The MEANS procedure is an excellent procedure for requesting summary statistics. This procedure can reproduce the following R functions: Mean(), Median(), Mode(), Range(), Var(), sd(), Sum(), Min(), Max(), and Quantile(). PROC MEANS will apply the function to the entire variable. So if we take the mean of the variable, it will take the mean of the entire column vector.

As shown in the following syntax, in the VAR statement of the MEANS procedure, we specify all the variables we want to use:

**PROC MEANS DATA=***SAS-data-set <options>*;
    **VAR** *variable-1 … variable-n*;
**RUN;**

Program 5.7 shows an example using the cars data set and MPG city and MPG highway. If we run this procedure in Program 5.7, we get the default output. Specifically, it would reproduce the Mean, Standard Deviation, Min, and Max function. And it would also give the number observations used to estimate those values.

**Program 5.7: PROC MEANS**

```
proc means data=sp4r.cars maxdec=2;
    var mpg_city mpg_highway;
run;
```

**Output 5.7: Results of Program 5.7**

| Variable | N | Mean | Std Dev | Minimum | Maximum |
|----------|-----|-------|---------|---------|---------|
| MPG_City | 428 | 20.06 | 5.24 | 10.00 | 60.00 |
| MPG_Highway | 428 | 26.84 | 5.74 | 12.00 | 66.00 |

As you can see in Output 5.7, MPG City Mean is 20.06, the Standard Deviation is 5.24, and so on. The maxdec=2 option in the PROC MEANS statement makes everything a maximum of two decimal places. Otherwise, you can get more decimal places than you need.

There are many different options to customize the output in a PROC MEANS procedure. You can generate all these descriptive statistics with these keywords shown in Table 5.2. You can specify Confidence Limits (CLM), the RANGE, the SKEWNESS of the distribution, the Variance (VAR), the Standard Error (STDERR), and so on. You can also request percentiles with these pre-determined keywords.

**Table 5.2: PROC MEANS Statement Options**

| Descriptive Statistic Keywords | | | | |
|------|------|----------|--------|--------|
| CLM | CSS | CV | LCLM | MAX |
| MEAN | MIN | MODE | N | NMISS |
| KURTOSIS | RANGE | SKEWNESS | STDDEV | STDERR |
| SUM | SUMWGT | UCLM | USS | VAR |

| Quantile Statistic Keywords | | | | |
|-------------|-----|-----|------|---------|
| MEDIAN | P50 | P1 | P5 | P10 | Q1 | P25 |
| Q3 | P75 | P90 | P95 | P99 | QRANGE |

For example, you can request the first percentile with the P1 keyword, the fifth percentile with the P5 keyword, and so on. Again, these are predefined, so you cannot simply say P15 to get the 15th percentile. But later you will learn how to request your own percentiles.

To customize the MEANS procedure output, simply tack on options to the MEANS procedure statement as shown in Program 5.8. In Program 5.8, we are requesting only the mean, median, and var options, which is going to give us the mean, median, and variance in the table shown in Output 5.8. It's not going to print the other default output.

**Program 5.8: PROC MEANS with Options**

```
proc means data=sp4r.cars maxdec=2 mean median var;
    var mpg_city mpg_highway;
run;
```

**Output 5.8: Results of Program 5.8**

| Variable | Mean | Median | Variance |
|---|---|---|---|
| MPG_City | 20.06 | 19.00 | 27.44 |
| MPG_Highway | 26.84 | 26.00 | 32.96 |

## PROC UNIVARIATE

The final procedure that we will talk about in this section is the UNIVARIATE procedure. You can generate lots of different output with this procedure, more than we can cover in this section.

You can generate moments like means, skewness, kurtosis. You can generate basic statistical measures, for example, mean, median, standard deviation. You can do testing for location. It gives you predefined quantiles by default, and it also prints the extreme observations—the five highest and lowest observations of the variable. Some example output from PROC UNIVARIATE is shown in Figure 5.2.

**Figure 5.2: Example PROC UNIVARIATE Output**

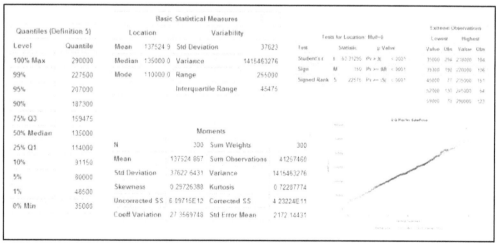

The UNIVARIATE procedure is used same way as the MEANS procedure. Just list all the variables you want to use in the VAR statement as shown in the following syntax:

**PROC UNIVARIATE DATA=**SAS-data-set <options>;
   **VAR** variable-1 … variable-n;
**RUN;**

You can also generate some graphics in PROC UNIVARIATE. For example, you can use the HISTOGRAM statement similarly to PROC SGPLOT to create a histogram. You can also generate a QQ Plot directly in the UNIVARIATE procedure using the QQPLOT statements syntax as follows:

**HISTOGRAM** variable-1 … variable-n / <options>;
**QQPLOT** variable-1 … variable-n / <options>;

For examples of how to use PROC UNIVARIATE, see the SAS documentation. We will also discuss how to control the output of this procedure in the next section.

# Output Delivery System

In this section, you will learn how to customize your PROC step output, specifically, how to return only specific tables and graphics and create new tables from PROC step results.

In R, we typically create a model object and then print the default output. We can also pull fields from the object, like the names, or the residuals, and so on. Then we can create data frames from those fields as shown in Figure 5.3. In this section, the SAS equivalent is pulling fields from an object to customize your results.

**Figure 5.3: R Script**

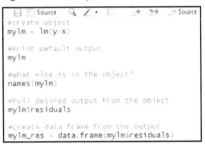

First, to customize our results in SAS, we need to talk about the Output Delivery System (ODS). SAS procedures and DATA steps simply produce raw data. For example, when we run the CORR procedure, we get the output shown in Figure 5.4. But PROC CORR only produces the raw data for the table cells, in this case, 1.00000, 0.63080, 0.38155, and so on. It's the Output Delivery System that actually provides structure to the table, the color, titles, headings, and so on.

**Figure 5.4: PROC CORR Output**

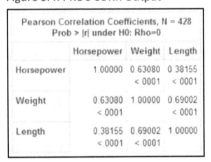

Why is this important?

Well, we can actually get inside the Output Delivery System and alter the appearance of the output, for example, the style, color, font, and so on. We can also change the destination file type of the output. In this section, you will learn how to select specific output and also create new data tables from that output.

## Customizing Output with the ODS SELECT Statement

PROC UNIVARIATE produces a lot of default output. For example, it produces the Quantiles table, the Moments table, the QQ Plot graphic, and so on. Maybe we don't actually want to print all this material. Maybe we only want to print the Basic Statistical Measures table and the QQ Plot graphic. How can we customize these results?

To do this, we use the ODS SELECT statement *before* running the procedure. Then specify the object name, specifically the table or graphic name, and SAS will only print those tables or graphics to the results page as shown in the following syntax:

**ODS SELECT** *object-name-1 ... object-name-n*;

You can specify as many tables and graphics as you want in a single ODS SELECT statement.

> **Tip:** This is identical to using the $ symbol in R to pull output from an object.

One way to determine what the table and graphic names are is to use the ODS TRACE ON statement. When we run this statement, any output that is generated to the results page, the tables and graphic names, are printed to the log as shown in Program 5.9 and Output 5.9.

**Program 5.9: ODS TRACE Statement**

```
odstrace on;

proc univariate data=ameshousing;
    varsaleprice;
    qqplotsaleprice/normal(mu=estsigma=est);
run;

odstrace off;
```

**Output 5.9: Log of Program 5.9**

```
Output Added
..............
Name:       Moments
Label:      Moments
Template:   base.univariate.Moments
Path:       Univariate.SalePrice.Moments
..............

Output Added:
..............
Name:       BasicMeasures
Label:      Basic Measures of Location and Variability
Template:   base.univariate.Measures
Path:       Univariate.SalePrice.BasicMeasures
..............

Output Added:
..............
Name:       TestsForLocation
Label:      Tests For Location
Template:   base.univariate.Location
Path:       Univariate.SalePrice.TestsForLocation
..............

Output Added:
..............
Name:       Quantiles
Label:      Quantiles
Template:   base.univariate.Quantiles
Path:       Univariate.SalePrice.Quantiles
..............

Output Added:
..............
Name:       ExtremeObs
Label:      Extreme Observations
Template:   base.univariate.ExtObs
Path:       Univariate.SalePrice.ExtremeObs
..............
```

```
Output Added:
..............
Name:       QQPlot
Label:      Panel 1
Template:   base.univariate.Graphics.QQPlot
Path:       Univariate.SalePrice.QQPlot.QQPlot
..............
```

Then we can grab those table and graphics names from the log and use ODS SELECT to customize the output by printing only the BasicMeasures table and QQ plot in the next run as shown in Program 5.10 and Output 5.10.

**Program 5.10: ODS SELECT Statement**

```
ods select basicmeasures qqplot;

proc univariate data=sp4r.ameshousing;
    var saleprice;
    qqplot saleprice / normal(mu=est sigma=est);
run;
```

**Output 5.10: Results of Program 5.10**

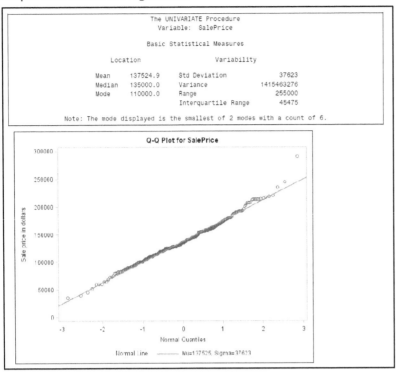

If you don't want to keep printing all this output to the log, simply use the ODS TRACE OFF statement after.

## Saving Results with the ODS OUTPUT Statement

Next, we will use the Output Delivery System to create new data tables from the PROC STEP results tables and choose specific summary statistics to include in the tables. Perhaps when you ran the UNIVARIATE procedure in Program 5.10 and generated the Basic Statistical Measures table, you also wanted to save it as a new SAS data set. To save an output table as a SAS data set, we will use the ODS OUTPUT statement prior to running our procedure as shown in the following syntax:

**ODS OUTPUT** *output-object-name* = *data-set-name*;

In the ODS OUTPUT statement you will first specify the object name, which is the same table name that we used in ODS SELECT. Then you will set that table name equal to a new SAS data set name. For example, in Program 5.11, our new table name will be SP_BasicMeasures. SP is going to be for sale price, the variable that we are analyzing in the UNIVARIATE procedure.

**Program 5.11: ODS OUTPUT Statement**

```
ods output basicmeasures = SP_BasicMeasures;

proc univariate data=ameshousing;
    var saleprice;
run;
```

If you are familiar with R, then it looks a little bit peculiar that the new data set name is on the right side of the assignment statement and the object name is on the left, but just be aware that that is the syntax in SAS. You can specify as many object names equal to data set names as you would like in a single ODS OUTPUT statement. After you finish your ODS OUTPUT statement, then run the appropriate procedure to generate the table and save it.

## Saving Results with the OUTPUT Statement

What if you don't want to save the entire table? What if all you want to do is save a single summary statistic, like the mean? It might not make sense to only save one summary statistic to an entire data table, but in the next section, you will see a good reason why you would want to do it. To save a single summary statistic, use the OUTPUT statement (not to be confused with the ODS OUTPUT statement) to customize the new data table. The OUTPUT statement enables the user to select which individual values from the results tables to place in the new data table. This avoids keeping unwanted statistics from default results tables. Immediately following the OUTPUT statement, use the OUT equal to option, and specify a new SAS data set name as shown in the following syntax:

**OUTPUT OUT=**_new-data-set-namekeyword-1= variable-name-1… keyword-n= variable-name-n_;

For example, in Program 5.12, we use the OUTPUT statement to create a new table called stats.

**Program 5.12: OUTPUT Statement**
```
procunivariate data=ameshousing;
    varsaleprice;
    output out=stats mean=sp_mean;
run;
```

Program 5.12 uses the keyword mean to save the mean. You can find more keywords listed on the SAS documentation page. We set the SAS data set variable name equal to sp_mean. You can request as many summary statistics as there are keywords in the OUTPUT statement.

We will see the OUTPUT statement in a later chapter when we get into modeling. For example, we will save residuals and predicted values, and then generate residual-by-predicted plots with those new SAS data sets.

## Creating Macro Variables

By this point, you have probably noticed that the scope of the variables in SAS are exclusive to the data set they were created in. For example, if we create a new data set called myvars and specify mymean and mysd as two numeric values, we cannot then use them in other DATA or PROC steps with a different data set. For example, we cannot go into the test data set and standardize the value y with mymean and mysd from the myvars data set. Likewise, we cannot use mymean in the PRINT procedure when we use a different data set as well.

How can we circumvent this problem in SAS? In R, we would just create the new variables. For example, mymean and mysd are just numeric values that we could use to standardize value y as shown in Figure 5.5.

**Figure 5.5: R Script**

This section shows you how to replicate this process manually in SAS. You will also learn how to automate the process. What if your data changes? You do not want to have to type out 123.45. You just want to take the mean of y and the standard deviation of y then use it to standardize values.

### Manually Create a Macro Variable

In this section, you will learn an easy way to manually create a macro variable. Then we will automate the process using the SQL procedure.

To create this variable like you would in R, in SAS you will create a macro variable with the %LET statement. Specify the new variable name and just set it equal to whatever value you want using the following syntax:

**%LET** _variable-name = value_;

Suppose you have a numeric variable, for example, height=67. To create the variable height=67, simply use the %LET statement and set height equal to 67 as follows:

```
%let height=67;
```

To create a character macro variable, you will use the exact same syntax with the %LET statement. Because macro variables are stored as text, the same syntax is used for both numeric and character macro variables. We will call this macro variable name and set it equal to Jordan Bakerman.

```
%let name = Jordan Bakerman;
```

Notice that we do not use quotation marks like we would in R. SAS stores everything as a text string, so we do not need to quote anything. If you do add quotation marks, the quotation marks are going to be saved inside the macro variable as part of the text string. SAS also saves the capitalization of J and B in the macro variable. Whatever you type in is going to be saved exactly as-is.

Let's look at some of the following characteristics of macro variables:

- Number tokens are stored as text strings.
- The minimum length is 0 characters (null value).
- The maximum length is 64k characters.
- Case is preserved.
- Leading and trailing blanks are removed.
- Quotation marks are stored as part of the value.

## Using Macro Variables

Now that we know how to create a macro variable, how do we use it? Macro variable references begin with an ampersand followed by the macro variable name as shown in the following syntax:

**&myvar**

Imagine we have the variable myvar. To use it inside a DATA or PROC step, or wherever you want, say &myvar. Then when you run the script, it is going to resolve to the variable that you have specified.

Macro variable references are also called symbolic references, but we will refer to them simply as macro variable references. Here are some other qualities of macro variable references:

- They can appear anywhere in a program so that you can use them in any DATA or PROC step that you want. When you use the %LET statement, the macro variable is global.
- The macro variable name is not case sensitive. For example, myvar is not case sensitive. But the values that you have stored in that variable are case sensitive.
- They are passed to the macro processor to be resolved by SAS. So &myvar will resolve to whatever you specified.

## Examples

Let's look at a few examples of using a macro variable. In the first example, we will use the PRINT procedure in Program 5.13.

**Program 5.13: Code Without a Macro Variable**

```
proc print data=ameshousing;
    where yr_sold = 2010;
    var yr_sold saleprice;
    title "Price of Homes Sold in 2010";
run;
```

**Output 5.13: Partial Results of Program 5.13**

```
   Price of Homes Sold in 2010

Obs          Yr_Sold       SalePrice

1               2010          213500
2               2010          191500
3               2010          115000
```

Notice in Program 5.13 there are two instances of the year 2010—one in the WHERE statement and one in the TITLE statement. Of course, you can imagine we might have much more code where we want to change the value 2010 several times—even 10, 20, or 30 times. This is just a small example.

So how would update Program 5.13 to use a macro variable to change 2010 in both instances easily? First, use the %LET statement to create a new macro variable called year and let it equal 2010. Now, as you can see in Program 5.14, we can replace all instances of 2010 in the PRINT procedure with &year in the WHERE statement and the TITLE statement.

**Program 5.14: Macro Variable**

```
%let year = 2010;

proc print data=ameshousing;
    where yr_sold = &year;
    var yr_sold saleprice;
    title "Price of Homes Sold in &year";
run;
```

If you run Program 5.14, the output will be identical to Output 5.13.

But what if you wanted to change the year to 2011, 2012, and so on? Simply change the macro variable in the %LET statement. That way you don't have to change it in every spot of the PRINT procedure.

Let's look at another example using character data.

**Program 5.15: Code Without Macro Variable**

```
proc print data=ameshousing;
    where garage_type_2 = "Attached";
    var yr_sold saleprice;
    title "Homes Sold with Attached Garage";
run;
```

**Output 5.15: Partial Results of Program 5.15**

```
  Homes Sold with Attached Garage

Obs          Yr_Sold       SalePrice

1               2010          213500
2               2010          191500
4               2010          160000
```

In Program 5.15 we are running the PRINT procedure again, but you will notice this time in the WHERE statement, we are using garage_type_2. That variable is either Attached or Detached. Because we are specifying character data in the WHERE statement, we need to quote the value Attached. Notice also the word Attached is in the TITLE statement.

How can we use a macro variable to make it easier to change that value? The %LET statement, of course. Let's create a new macro variable called gtype and let it be equal to Attached as shown in Program 5.16. It is very important that you keep the A capitalized because that is how it appears in your data set. Then supply the gtype macro variable into the PRINT procedure where the word Attached was, as well as in the WHERE and TITLE statement.

**Program 5.16: Macro Variable**

```
%let gtype = Attached;

proc print data=ameshousing;
    where garage_type_2 = "&gtype";
    var yr_sold saleprice;
    title "Homes Sold with &gtype Garage";
run;
```

It's extremely important when you are quoting a macro variable to use double quotation marks. Why? Because this allows the macro variable to resolve. &gtype will resolve to the word Attached. If you used single quotation marks, it would leave it as &gtype. There is no value in your data set for garage_type_2 called &gtype. When in doubt when working with macro variables, use double quotation marks.

> **Tip:** You must use double quotation marks when you refer to a macro variable.

## Creating Global Macro Variables

In the previous section, we saw how to create macros variables manually with the %LET statement. Now let's automate the process using SQL and the following steps:

- **Step 1: Create a SAS data table**. In order to query a data set, we need to actually have a data set with useful information.

- **Step 2: Use PROC SQL to create a macro variable.** Use the following syntax:

```
PROC SQL;
    SELECT variable-name
    INTO :macro-variable-name
    FROM data-table-name;
```

### Step 1: Create a SAS Data Table

In Program 5.17, we run the MEANS procedure using the OUTPUT statement to create a new SAS data set with the values for mean and standard deviation. The variable names in this data set stats are going to be mean and sd.

**Program 5.17: Create SAS Data Table**

```
proc means data=ameshousing;
    var saleprice;
    output out=stats mean=mean std=sd;
run;
```

### Step 2: Use PROC SQL to Create a Macro Variable

Now we can query the data and create new macro variables. To do so, we will use PROC SQL. Start with the SELECT statement and specify the variable-name in the data set, in this case mean, as shown in Program 5.18. Use the keyword into, and the colon operator, and specify a new macro variable, sp_mean. Finally, tell it what data set to look at, stats. Likewise, select the standard deviation and put that into a new macro variable called sp_sd, again, from the stats data set.

**Program 5.18: PROC SQL**

```
proc sql;
    select mean into :sp_mean from stats;
    select sd into :sp_sd from stats;
quit;
```

Just like the %LET statement that we used when creating a macro variable manually, these macro variables are also global. You can use them in any data or PROC steps that you would like.

## %PUT Statement

If you create a macro variable automatically, and perhaps put your program away for a week or two, when you come back, to remind yourself of what you have done, you can use the %PUT statement to write a nice message to yourself in the log using the following syntax:

**%PUT** *text*;

In this case, let's remind ourselves that the mean and standard deviation of the sale price variable is &sp_mean and &sp_sd. When you run this %PUT statement in Program 5.19, it's going to print that text and resolve the macro variables.

**Program 5.18: %PUT Statement**

```
%put The mean and sd of the Sale Price
variable is &sp_mean and &sp_sd;
```

**Output 5.18: Log of Program 5.18**

```
The mean and sd of the Sale Price variable is
137524.87 and 37622.64
```

Writing a message to the log is an easy way to remind yourself what program you created. Quotation marks are not required in your %PUT statement. It will print it as is. And the %PUT statement is valid in open code on its own line. You do not need to include it in a DATA or PROC step.

## _USER_ Argument

Another useful piece of syntax in SAS is the _USER_ argument in the %PUT statement that uses the following syntax:

**%PUT** _USER_;

That piece of code prints all the macro variables that you have created in your current SAS session. In this chapter, we have created the GTYPE, YEAR, SP_MEAN, and SP_SD macro variables thus far, so those would be printed in the log.

You could also use the argument _ALL_ to see the included built-in SAS macro variables as well.

## Automatic Macro Variables

The built-in macro variables in SAS are called automatic macro variables. Visit the online SAS documentation page to view all of them. Table 5.3 shows just a small subset of the long list of automatic macro variables.

**Table 5.3: Selected Automatic Macro Variables**

| Name | Description |
|---|---|
| **SYSDATE** | Date of SAS invocation (06JAN14) |
| **SYSDATE9** | Date of SAS invocation (06JAN2014) |
| **SYSDAY** | Day of the week of SAS invocation (Friday) |
| **SYSTIME** | Time of SAS invocation (10:47) |
| **SYSSCP** | Operating system abbreviation (WIN, OS, HP 64) |
| **SYSVER** | Release of SAS software (9.3) |
| **SYSUSERID** | Login or user ID of current SAS process |

For example, if you wanted to know the day of the week, you would use the automatic macro variable SYSDAY. It would print the day of the week, in this case, Friday. If you want to print the date with a width of nine, you could use SYSDATE9, and so on. We will use a couple of automatic macro variables later in this book when we do some conditional processing.

> **Tip:** The macro variables **SYSDATE**, **SYSDATE9**, and **SYSTIME** store text, not SAS date or time values.

## Creating Macro Programs

In this section, you will learn how to create a macro program in order to run SAS code repetitively. We can also run SAS DATA and PROC steps conditionally or iteratively.

Think of a macro program simply as an R function to provide whatever customization you want. For example, in Figure 5.6 we are creating a macro program called randnorm and passing it a single parameter. It's simply the number of observations we are going to simulate from a normal distribution. And then we will use that data set to generate some reports. For example, in Figure 5.6, we want a table and graphic. We do all of this inside a single program. Of course, once you type this R function up once, you can use the function and pass it whatever parameter you want. In Figure 5.6, we change n to be 10,000.

**Figure 5.6: R Script**

```
      Source on Save                      Run        Source
#Create a Function
randnorm = function(n){

  #Generate Data
  vec = rnorm(n)

  #Print Summary Statistics
  mean(vec)
  median(vec)
  sd(vec)
  min(vec)
  max(vec)

  #Create Plots
  par(mfrow=c(1,2))
  hist(vec)
  plot(vec,type="b")
}

#Use Function and Change Parameters
randnorm(n=10000)
```

By the end of this section, you should be able to write a program like this in SAS. To do this in SAS, we will need to use a DATA step to generate the data, PROC MEANs to print some summary statistics, and PROC SGPLOT to create the plots. So in SAS, we are going to be combining lots of different DATA and PROC steps in one single macro program—or, again, think of it as an R function.

The macro facility is a text processing facility for automating and customizing the generation of SAS code. You should be thinking, "What code do I actually want to generate and compile inside my macro program?" The macro facility minimizes the amount of code that you need to enter.

The macro facility supports the following:

- Symbolic substitution within SAS code. For example, we can pass it a macro variable or parameters.

- Automated production of SAS code. We can run an unsupervised script.

- Conditional construction of SAS code. We can generate certain code, plots, or reports, depending on whatever parameters we pass the macro.

## Defining a Macro

So how do we actually create a macro? We are going to use %MACRO to start and %MEND to end as shown in the following syntax:

**%MACRO** *macro-name*;
  *macro-text*
**%MEND** *<macro-name>*;

In Program 5.19, we use the %MACRO to start and then name the macro today. Anything between %MACRO and %MEND will be the programming statements. In this program we have %put, so all this macro does is write a message to the log.

**Program 5.19: Defining a Macro**

```
%macro today;
    %put Today is &sysday &sysdate9;
%mend;
```

> **Tip:** Macro names follow SAS naming conventions and cannot be reserved names such as names of macro statements or functions (for example, LET and SCAN).

## Calling a Macro

After the macro is compiled, the macro is stored in the Work library with the name sasmacr. To call the macro variable, we will simply tack on a percent sign to the macro name as shown in the following syntax:

*%macro-name*

To run the today macro created in Program 5.19, simply use the name with the percent sign as shown in Program 5.20.

**Program 5.20: Macro Call**

```
%today
```

**Output 5.20: Log of Program 5.20**

```
178 %today
Today is Friday 01JAN2016
```

When we Program 5.20, it is going to run the %PUT statement within the macro. Therefore, it generates to the log the message that today is Friday, 01 January, 2016—or whatever day it happens to be when you run the program.

A macro call can appear anywhere in code. It does not have to be in a DATA or PROC step. It can just be on its own line. It's passed to the macro processor, so it can run the statements inside the macro. It's not a statement. You do not need to use a semi-colon after you call the macro. Notice there is no semi-colon after %today in Program 5.20. It runs just as it is.

## Customizing with Parameter Lists

A parameter list is a list of macro variables referenced within the macro. There are three types of parameter lists:

1. positional – must appear in the same order as their corresponding parameter names
2. keyword – assigned a default value after an equal sign
3. mixed – has both positional parameters and keyword parameters

Just like in R, we can pass macros a parameter list to customize the program even further. And just like in R, we can use positional keyword or a mixture of those parameter lists. In R, you probably don't know the exact names of the parameters. You have probably just bypassed that part. But in SAS, there is more structure, so you need to be more aware of what a positional and keyword parameter is.

## Positional Parameters

In Program 5.21 we are creating a macro called calc. Notice that it is just the MEANS procedure. There are two positional parameters—DSN for Data Set Name separated by a comma and vars for the variables that we are going to put in the VAR statement.

**Program 5.21: Creating a Macro with Positional Parameters**

```
%macro calc(dsn,vars);
    proc means data=&dsn;
        var &vars;
    run;
%mend calc;

%calc(business,yield)
```

Notice that when we pass in those parameters, we are passing them in as if they are macro variables. We are tacking on an ampersand to DSN and vars in the MEANS procedure.

When we call the macro with %calc, we simply list the data set name—in this case, business—and the variables—in this case, just yield.

Why are these positional parameters? Well, the parameter values must appear in the same order as their corresponding parameter names. So the first argument in the macro call of %calc—business—has to correspond to the first parameter in the macro definition—in this case, DSN. The same can be said for the second argument. Yield must correspond to vars.

## Keyword Parameters

Keyword parameters, on the other hand, are assigned a default value after an equal sign. In Program 5.22, we are creating a macro program called count, which is simply the FREQ procedure.

**Program 5.22: Creating a Macro with Keyword Parameters**

```
%macro count(opts=,start=01jan08,stop=31dec08);
    proc freq data=orion.orders;
        where order_date between
            "&start" and "&stop";
        table order_type / &opts;
        title1 "Orders from &start to &stop";
    run;
%mend count;
```

Notice in Program 5.22 there are three keyword parameters—opts equal to the null value, start equal to 01jan08, and stop equal to the 31st of December, '08. In the FREQ procedure, we use those dates in the WHERE statement to provide condition. In the TABLE statement after the forward slash, we provide the opts as the keyword parameter. So all three parameters have a default value.

The first parameter has a null value by default. On the final call, all parameters receive their default value. The empty parentheses are important because this macro "knows" that it has a parameter list. If you omit the parentheses, the macro does not execute but patiently waits for its expected parameter list. If the next token submitted does not begin a parameter list, the macro "knows" that a parameter list is not forthcoming and executes using default parameter values. Parentheses, even if empty, are recommended as explicit and unambiguous, and they guarantee immediate execution of the macro.

So how do we call the macro when we are using keyword parameters? A few different ways are shown in Program 5.23.

**Program 5.23: Call a Macro with Keyword Parameters**

```
options mprint;
%count(opts=nocum) ❶
%count(stop=01jul08,opts=nocum nopercent) ❷
%count() ❸
```

❶ The first way is to run %count with just a single keyword parameter—opts equal to nocum. And then the other two keyword parameters just stick to their default values.

❷ A second way to call the macro is to change the order of the keyword parameters as they are listed in the macro definition. So first, we start with stop equal to changing the date. Then we specify the options NOCUM and NOPERCENT. Keyword parameters can be out of order, whereas positional parameters cannot.

Also, if you want to change the keyword parameter in the macro call, you have to use the keyword parameter name and set it equal to a new value. For example, you cannot just say nocum. It will not default to the first parameter opts. You have to literally say opts equal to nocum.

❸ And finally, if you run %count with empty parentheses, it will just default to the parameters in the macro definition.

## Mixed Parameters

In a mixed parameter list, we have both positional parameters and keyword parameters. You are required to list the positional parameters first in the macro definition followed by the keyword parameters. The same is true for the macro call, as shown in Program 5.24.

**Program 5.24: Creating and Calling a Macro with Mixed Parameters**

```
%macro count(opts,start=01jan08,stop=31dec08);  ❶
    proc freq data=orion.orders;
        where order_date between
            "&start" and "&stop";
        table order_type / &opts;
        title1 "Orders from &start to &stop";
    run;
%mend count;
options mprint;
%count(nocum)  ❷
%count(stop=30jun08,start=01apr08)  ❸
%count(nocum nopercent,stop=30jun08) ❹
%count() ❺
```

❶ Notice in the %MACRO statement, opts is now a positional parameter. We are not setting it equal to the null value. But we are leaving start and stop as keyword parameters.

❷ In our first macro call of %count, we are only changing the positional parameter opts to nocum. Start and stop keyword parameters will be at their default values.

❸ In the second macro call, we are changing the stop and start keyword parameters to two different dates. Notice that we have not specified anything for the positional parameter opts. If we do not change the positional parameter, it defaults to the null value.

❹ In the third macro call, notice we have changed both the opts positional parameter and the stop keyword parameter. This is important. The positional parameter must come first. So we have to change opts to nocum and nopercent, and then we can change the keyword parameters—in this case, stop.

❺ In the final macro call, we will run it with the null value. opts will default to the null value. And both start and stop keyword parameters will be left at their default values.

# Macro Statements: An Example

A macro language statement instructs the macro processor to perform an operation. It consists of a keyword and begins with the percent sign, just like our macro call and macro definition, and ends in a semicolon. Macro statements enable the following actions:

- **conditional processing** – choose which PROC or DATA steps to run based on certain parameters

- **parameter validation** – check if a value is outside a specific range, and if it is, tell SAS to throw an error so that it doesn't keep processing

- **iterative processing** – use loops to create a dynamic program that executes for a number of iterations based on some conditions

For more information, look up macro statements on the online documentation page. There are many different macro statements that you can incorporate into your own macro programming.

This example will focus on iterative processing. We want to read in multiple CSV files in a single macro program so that we don't have to keep typing out PROC IMPORT or the appropriate DATA steps. This is one instance where macro programming can help quite a bit.

For example, imagine you work in a business where a daily sales report is generated every night. Every Friday, a weekly report is generated. Let's determine the best method to automate both of these reports.

For the daily report, we want to create a macro program that runs a PRINT procedure. But if it is Friday, we also want the macro program to generate the MEANS procedure.

What are a few different ways that we could accomplish this? In this example, we will look at two different methods, but you could probably come up with several more solutions of your own.

- **Method 1:** We will create multiple macros, including a driver macro, meaning the driver macro will call the appropriate macro conditionally where necessary.

- **Method 2:** We will create a single macro and use macro statements like %DO and %END to run SAS syntax conditionally.

## Method 1

First, let's create separate macros for the daily and weekly programs. The daily macro program will simply be the PRINT procedure shown in Program 5.25. Likewise, the weekly macro program will be the MEANS procedure.

**Program 5.25: Method 1 – Separate Macros**

```
%macro daily;
    proc print data=orion.order_fact;
        where order_date="&sysdate9";
        var product_id total_retail_price;
        title "Daily sales: &sysdate9";
    run;
%mend daily;

%macro weekly;
    proc means data=orion.order_fact n sum mean;
        where order_date between
            "&sysdate9"-6 and "&sysdate9";
        var quantity total_retail_price;
        title "Weekly sales: &sysdate9";
    run;
%mend weekly;

%macro reports;
    %daily
    %if &sysday=Friday %then %weekly;
%mend reports;
```

Notice in Program 5.25 that we created a DRIVER macro called REPORTS that always calls the daily macro and conditionally calls the weekly macro. Program 5.25 is a true macro program, with a macro call and a macro language statement. This is a "system-driven" macro insofar as it is driven by or makes a decision according to system information, such as the day of the week.

In order to conditionally run the weekly macro, we need to use macro statements. A lot of the macro statements are very similar to what we have seen in SAS syntax already. The only difference in the macro programming language, is that we will tack on a percent sign. So notice we use %IF and provide it an expression. If our automatic macro variable SYSDAY is equal to Friday, we use %THEN and then run the weekly macro that uses the MEANS procedure. Use the following syntax within macro statements:

**%IF** *expression* **%THEN** *action*;
**%ELSE** *action*;

Table 5.4 shows some of the differences between macro expressions and SAS expressions. For example, in macro expressions, character constants are not quoted or case-sensitive. The %ELSE statement is optional and %IF-%THEN and %ELSE statements can be used inside a macro definition only.

**Table 5.4: Macro Expressions**

| | Macro Expressions | SAS Expressions |
|---|:---:|:---:|
| Arithmetic operators | ✓ | ✓ |
| Logical operators (Do not precede AND or OR with %.) | ✓ | ✓ |
| Comparison operators (symbols and mnemonics) | ✓ | ✓ |
| Case sensitivity | ✓ | ✓ |
| Special WHERE operators | | |
| Quotation marks | | ✓ |
| Ranges such as 1<=x<=10 | | ✓ |
| IN operator: parentheses required | | ✓ |

## Method 2

Program 5.26 shows an alternative method to accomplish the same goal. Here we put everything in a single macro instead of creating three separate macros. We are creating the macro reports, and if we run reports, we automatically want it to execute the PRINT procedure. Again, we want to use macro statements to tell SAS to conditionally run the MEANS procedure. The %DO %END syntax enables users to write multiple statements between the %DO and %END. This is useful for conditionally running DATA or PROC steps.

**Program 5.26: Method 2 – Single Macro**

```
%macro reports;
    proc print data=orion.order_fact;
        where order_date="&sysdate9";
        var product_id total_retail_price;
        title "Daily sales: &sysdate9";
    run;
%if &sysday=Friday %then %do;
    proc means data=orion.order_fact n sum mean;
        where order_date between
            "&sysdate9"d - 6 and "&sysdate9"d;
        var quantity total_retail_price;
        title "Weekly sales: &sysdate9";
```

```
   run;
 %end;
%mend reports;
```

In Program 5.26 we have an entire PROC step, so we need to use a DO group. If it is true, then the program runs the MEANS procedure. Don't forget the %END statement! Now when we run the report's macro, it will automatically run the PRINT procedure and conditionally run the MEANS procedure. Everything is under one roof.

# Exercises

1.  Which SAS procedures are used to reproduce the R functions min(), cov(), table(), and sd()?

    a.  FREQ, MEANS, CORR, MEANS

    b.  MEANS, CORR, FREQ, MEANS

    c.  MEANS FREQ, CORR, MEANS

    d.  CORR, FREQ, FREQ, MEANS

2.  Which statements are true regarding macro variables? Select all that apply.

    a.  Macro variables must be assigned in a DATA or PROC step.

    b.  Case is preserved.

    c.  To reference a macro variable, you must use the & symbol.

    d.  Macro variables can be used only three times or less in a PROC step.

3.  The SAS code below creates the PROC CORR and PROC MEANS analyses.

    ```
    %let cont_var = saleprice garage_area basement_area gr_liv_area;

    ods select pearsoncorr;
    proc corr data=sp4r.ameshousing;
       var cont_var;
    run;

    proc means data=sp4r.ameshousing;
       var cont_var;
    run;
    ```

    a.  True

    b.  False

1.  Navigate to the TABLES statement on the SAS documentation page for the FREQ procedure. What does the PROC step below do?

    ```
    proc freq data=sp4r.cars;
        tables origin*type / chisq;
    run;
    ```

2.  What types of functions do you make in R that call R functions and packages? How can this be translated into SAS PROC and DATA steps?

3.  There are three mistakes in the SAS code below. Can you find all three?

    ```
    %macro test(condition=50000,dt);
        proc means data=dt;
            where msrp > &condition;
        run;
    %mend;
    %test(cars,100000)
    ```

Use the AmesHousing data set to complete Exercises 1, 2, 3, and 5. Use the Cars data set to complete Exercise 4.

1.  **Using Descriptive Procedures and ODS**

    a.  Navigate to the SAS Help documentation and view the TABLES statement options for the FREQ procedure. Which option enables you to create a frequency plot? Use PROC FREQ to create one-way frequency tables for the variables **central_air** and **house_style** along with frequency plots.

What percentage of homes in this sample have central air? What percent are only one story?

The FREQ Procedure

| Central_ Air | Frequency | Percent | Cumulative Frequency | Cumulative Percent |
|---|---|---|---|---|
| N | 42 | 14.00 | 42 | 14.00 |
| Y | 258 | 86.00 | 300 | 100.00 |

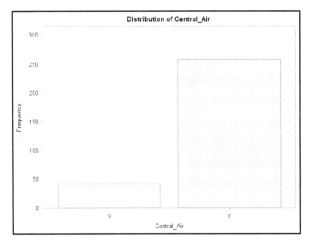

| House_ Style | Frequency | Percent | Cumulative Frequency | Cumulative Percent |
|---|---|---|---|---|
| 1.5Fin | 28 | 9.33 | 28 | 9.33 |
| 1.5Unf | 4 | 1.33 | 32 | 10.67 |
| 1Story | 194 | 64.67 | 226 | 75.33 |
| 2.5Unf | 2 | 0.67 | 228 | 76.00 |
| 2Story | 38 | 12.67 | 266 | 88.67 |
| SFoyer | 13 | 4.33 | 279 | 93.00 |
| SLvl | 21 | 7.00 | 300 | 100.00 |

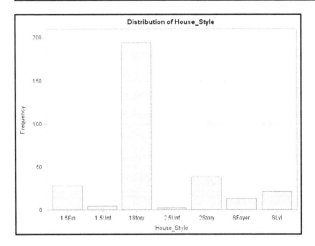

b.  The default PROC CORR output gives a table of simple statistics and correlation coefficients. Use ODS SELECT to print only the correlation coefficients for the variables **saleprice, garage_area, basement_area**, and **gr_liv_area**. (Hint: It might be easiest to use the ODS TRACE statement to learn the table name instead of going to the documentation page.) Is there a statistically significant correlation between **saleprice** and each of the other variables?

```
                              The CORR Procedure

                   Pearson Correlation Coefficients, N = 300
                         Prob > |r| under H0: Rho=0

                         Sale        Garage_      Basement_      Gr_Liv_
                        Price          Area          Area          Area
        SalePrice     1.00000        0.57892       0.68956       0.65046
                                      <.0001        <.0001        <.0001


        Garage_Area   0.57892        1.00000       0.35630       0.33283
                       <.0001                       <.0001        <.0001


        Basement_Area 0.68956        0.35630       1.00000       0.43985
                       <.0001         <.0001                      <.0001


        Gr_Liv_Area   0.65046        0.33283       0.43985       1.00000
                       <.0001         <.0001        <.0001
```

c.  Use PROC MEANS to print the 10th percentile, median, and 90th percentile for the variables **saleprice** and **gr_liv_area**. In addition, use the CLASS statement to separate the summary statistics by the **yr_sold** variable. Finally, save the output using ODS OUTPUT and name the table **summary_table**. Print the table to ensure it is saved. Which year had the highest median sale price?

```
                                  VName_       SalePrice_    SalePrice_    SalePrice_
      Obs      Yr_Sold    NObs    SalePrice        P10         Median         P90

       1         2006      55     SalePrice      93500        131000        169000
       2         2007      72     SalePrice      96500        128500        180500
       3         2008      62     SalePrice      87000        136250        181900
       4         2009      73     SalePrice      91300        144000        192000
       5         2010      38     SalePrice     100000        148875        192000

               VName_Gr_      Gr_Liv_Area_    Gr_Liv_Area_    Gr_Liv_Area_
      Obs      Liv_Area           P10           Median            P90

       1      Gr_Liv_Area        864            1092            1368
       2      Gr_Liv_Area        864            1076            1435
       3      Gr_Liv_Area        864            1185            1430
       4      Gr_Liv_Area        800            1210            1456
       5      Gr_Liv_Area        848           1146.5           1395
```

d.  Use PROC UNIVARIATE to analyze the **gr_liv_area** variable and create both a histogram and a QQPlot. For the histogram, overlay a normal and density kernel estimate. Use the OUTPUT statement to create a new data table of percentiles called **gr_percs**. Instead of providing the PCTLPTS= option a list, use the following syntax: `PCTLPTS= 40 to 60 by 2`. Let the prefixes for the saved percentiles be **gr_**. Print the table to ensure that it is saved.

```
 Obs    gr_40    gr_42    gr_44    gr_46    gr_48    gr_50    gr_52    gr_54    gr_56    gr_58    gr_60

  1    1063.5   1075.5   1087     1092    1109.5    1135     1151    1169.5    1191     1206     1218
```

2.  **Creating and Using a Macro Variable for Unsupervised Scripting**

    a.  Use the MEANS procedure to create a new data table with the median of the **SalePrice** variable.

    b.  Use PROC SQL to create a macro variable of the median **SalePrice** value.

    c.  In the **AmesHousing** data set, create a new variable that is a value of *1* if the **SalePrice** is greater than the median and *0* otherwise. Use PROC FREQ to create a frequency table of the new variable.

```
                          The FREQ Procedure

                                      Cumulative    Cumulative
      sp_bin    Frequency   Percent   Frequency      Percent

         0         153       51.00       153          51.00
         1         147       49.00       300         100.00
```

3. **Using the SYMPUTX Subroutine**

   a. The SYMPUTX subroutine enables you to create a macro variable inside a DATA step. Navigate to the online documentation for a complete description. Run the SAS code below (**SP4R05e03.sas**) and analyze both the code and log output. What does this code do?

   ```
   data _NULL_;
       x=-3;
       df=5;
       p=(1-probt(abs(x),df))*2;
       call symputx('sig_level',p);
   run;


   %put The significance level for the two-tailed t test is
        &sig_level;
   ```

   b. An alternative method to creating the macro variable in Exercise 2 is to use the SYMPUTX subroutine. Use a DATA _NULL_ step, a SET statement, and the SYMPUTX routine to create a macro variable for the median of the **saleprice** variable. Use the %PUT statement to ensure that the macro variable is created correctly.

4. **Creating a Macro to Generate Summary Statistics and Plots of Any Data Table**

   a. Open **SP4R05e04.sas**. Create the **mystats** macro. It should have a single positional parameter (**dt**) and four keyword parameters (**freq**=*no*, **means**=*no*, **opts**= , and **scatter**=*no*). Use the %IF, %THEN, and %END macro statements to validate the positional parameter. If no data table (**dt**) is supplied by the user, use %PUT to write the sentence "dt is a required argument" to the log and use the %RETURN statement to terminate the macro.

   b. Use PROC CONTENTS with the OUT= option to write the contents of the input data table (**dt**) to a new data table called **dtcontents**. Use PROC SQL to use the **Name** field from **dtcontents** to create two macro variables. Let **vars_cont** be the unique names of continuous variables in the data set separated by a space. Let **vars_cat** be the unique names of the categorical variables in the data set separated by a space.

   c. Use macro statements to generate a PROC FREQ step if the user supplied **freq**=*yes* when calling **mystats**. In this case, use PROC FREQ to create frequency tables for the categorical variables.

   d. Use macro statements to generate a PROC MEANS step if the user supplies **means**=*yes*. In this case, specify the continuous variables in the VAR statement. In addition, use the **opts** parameter in the PROC MEANS statement to easily change the descriptive statistics.

   e. Use macro statements to set a condition if the user supplies **scatter**=*yes*. In this case, use PROC SGSCATTER to create a scatter plot matrix of the continuous variables. End the creation of the macro with %MEND.

   f. Call the **mystats** macro to create frequency tables for the **cars** data set.

   ```
                         The FREQ Procedure

       Drive                      Cumulative    Cumulative
       Train    Frequency  Percent  Frequency     Percent

       All          92      21.50       92        21.50
       Front       226      52.80      318        74.30
       Rear        110      25.70      428       100.00

                                  Cumulative    Cumulative
       Make        Frequency  Percent  Frequency   Percent

       Acura          7       1.64        7        1.64
       Audi          19       4.44       26        6.07
       BMW           20       4.67       46       10.75
       Buick          9       2.10       55       12.85
       Cadillac       8       1.87       63       14.72
       Chevrolet     27       6.31       90       21.03
       Chrysler      15       3.50      105       24.53
       Dodge         13       3.04      118       27.57
       Ford          23       5.37      141       32.94
       GMC            8       1.87      149       34.81
       Honda         17       3.97      166       38.79
   ```

| | | | | |
|---|---|---|---|---|
| Hummer | 1 | 0.23 | 167 | 39.02 |
| Hyundai | 12 | 2.80 | 179 | 41.82 |
| Infiniti | 8 | 1.87 | 187 | 43.69 |
| Isuzu | 2 | 0.47 | 189 | 44.16 |
| Jaguar | 12 | 2.80 | 201 | 46.96 |
| Jeep | 3 | 0.70 | 204 | 47.66 |
| Kia | 11 | 2.57 | 215 | 50.23 |
| Land Rover | 3 | 0.70 | 218 | 50.93 |
| Lexus | 11 | 2.57 | 229 | 53.50 |
| Lincoln | 9 | 2.10 | 238 | 55.61 |
| MINI | 2 | 0.47 | 240 | 56.07 |
| Mazda | 11 | 2.57 | 251 | 58.64 |
| Mercedes-Benz | 26 | 6.07 | 277 | 64.72 |
| Mercury | 9 | 2.10 | 286 | 66.82 |
| Mitsubishi | 13 | 3.04 | 299 | 69.86 |
| Nissan | 17 | 3.97 | 316 | 73.83 |
| Oldsmobile | 3 | 0.70 | 319 | 74.53 |
| Pontiac | 11 | 2.57 | 330 | 77.10 |
| Porsche | 7 | 1.64 | 337 | 78.74 |
| Saab | 7 | 1.64 | 344 | 80.37 |
| Saturn | 8 | 1.87 | 352 | 82.24 |
| Scion | 2 | 0.47 | 354 | 82.71 |
| Subaru | 11 | 2.57 | 365 | 85.28 |
| Suzuki | 8 | 1.87 | 373 | 87.15 |
| Toyota | 28 | 6.54 | 401 | 93.69 |
| Volkswagen | 15 | 3.50 | 416 | 97.20 |
| Volvo | 12 | 2.80 | 428 | 100.00 |

**Partial Model Table**

The FREQ Procedure

| Model | Frequency | Percent | Cumulative Frequency | Cumulative Percent |
|---|---|---|---|---|
| 3.5 RL 4dr | 1 | 0.23 | 1 | 0.23 |
| 3.5 RL w/Navigation 4dr | 1 | 0.23 | 2 | 0.47 |
| 300M 4dr | 1 | 0.23 | 3 | 0.70 |
| 300M Special Edition 4dr | 1 | 0.23 | 4 | 0.93 |
| 325Ci 2dr | 1 | 0.23 | 5 | 1.17 |
| 325Ci convertible 2dr | 1 | 0.23 | 6 | 1.40 |

| Origin | Frequency | Percent | Cumulative Frequency | Cumulative Percent |
|---|---|---|---|---|
| Asia | 158 | 36.92 | 158 | 36.92 |
| Europe | 123 | 28.74 | 281 | 65.65 |
| USA | 147 | 34.35 | 428 | 100.00 |

| Type | Frequency | Percent | Cumulative Frequency | Cumulative Percent |
|---|---|---|---|---|
| Hybrid | 3 | 0.70 | 3 | 0.70 |
| SUV | 60 | 14.02 | 63 | 14.72 |
| Sedan | 262 | 61.21 | 325 | 75.93 |
| Sports | 49 | 11.45 | 374 | 87.38 |
| Truck | 24 | 5.61 | 398 | 92.99 |
| Wagon | 30 | 7.01 | 428 | 100.00 |

g.  Call the **mystats** macro to create the means output with `opts=mean median maxdec=2`. Generate a scatter plot matrix for the continuous variables.

The MEANS Procedure

| Variable | Label | Mean | Median |
|---|---|---|---|
| Cylinders | | 5.81 | 6.00 |
| EngineSize | Engine Size (L) | 3.20 | 3.00 |
| Horsepower | | 215.89 | 210.00 |
| Invoice | | 30014.70 | 25294.50 |
| Length | Length (IN) | 186.36 | 187.00 |
| MPG_City | MPG (City) | 20.06 | 19.00 |
| MPG_Highway | MPG (Highway) | 26.84 | 26.00 |
| MSRP | | 32774.86 | 27635.00 |
| Weight | Weight (LBS) | 3577.95 | 3474.50 |
| Wheelbase | Wheelbase (IN) | 108.15 | 107.00 |

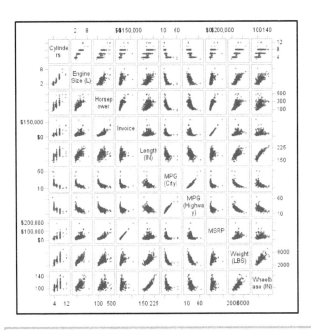

> **Tip**: A macro variable created inside a macro program is local in scope. For example, **vars_cont** and **vars_cat** can be referenced only inside the macro program. To create a global macro variable, you must use the SYMPUTX subroutine. The third argument enables the user to specify a global option for the macro variable that is being created. View the SAS online documentation for a complete description.

5. **Creating a Macro for Iterative Processing**

   Import a series of Excel workbook sheets into corresponding SAS data sets. The **amesbyyear** Excel workbook contains five separate sheets. Each sheet holds only the information for homes sold in a specific year. Each sheet is named according to the year (2006, 2007, 2008, 2009, 2010). The data begins on row 2, and row 1 contains all the variable names.

   a. Create a macro to iteratively call PROC IMPORT to read in each sheet of the **amesbyyear** spreadsheet. Call the macro **myimport** and give it two positional parameters (**firstyear**, **lastyear**). Let each new data set (one for each sheet) be named **year20##** where ## refers to each specific year.

   b. Call **myimport** to read in each sheet of the Excel file.

   > **Tip**: Remember that the iteration index value can be referenced as a macro variable.

   c. Check the **SP4R** library to ensure that all five data sets are created.

# Solutions

## Multiple Choice

1. b – The MEANS procedure can reproduce the min and sd functions, the covariance matrix is generated in the CORR procedure, and tables are created in the FREQ procedure.

2. b and c – Macro variables can be assigned in the %LET statement outside of DATA or PROC steps. Case is preserved for the text saved inside the macro variable however, the macro variable name is not case sensitive. To resolve the macro variable when you compile your code, you must use the & symbol.

3. b – Macro variables must be referenced with the & symbol.

## Short Answer

1. The CHISQ option requests chi-square tests of homogeneity or independence and measures of association that are based on the chi-square test statistic. The four summary statistics procedures in this section can also be used for conducting hypothesis tests by supplying specific options to the procedures.

2. Answers will be vast and vary; here is one possible response. Imagine you want to create a function that generates simple linear regression data for various values of the population intercept, slope, model error, and the number of sampled observations. You then want to fit the model with the simulated data to see the estimated parameters and a simple linear regression plot.

    In R, you would create a function with four parameters: intercept, slope, error, observations. You would then create a data frame with the observed values Y and covariates X. These would be created by simulating values with the random function rnorm(). You would then pass this data frame to the lm() function to fit the model and print results. Finally, you create a plot of Y by X with the plot() function and use the abline() function to add on a line of best fit. Each time you call this R function, you can create a new data set and see different results.

    To create an equivalent function in SAS, we will use a SAS macro program. To accomplish the same tasks, we will first create a data set with the values of Y and X using a DATA step and the RAND function. Next, we will use the REG procedure (discussed in chapter 6) to fit the model. Finally, we can use the SGPLOT procedure with the REG statement to plot the data and line of best fit. A macro program will automatically generate all the necessary code according to the parameters we pass it.

3. Since DT is a positional parameter, it must be referenced first in the macro definition.

    Macro parameters must be used as if they are macro variables. Thus, dt in the PROC MEANS statement must be referenced with the & symbol.

    To change the keyword parameter's default value in the macro call, you must use the parameter name.

```
%macro test(dt, condition=50000);
   proc means data=&dt;
      where msrp > &condition;
   run;
%mend;
%test(cars,condition=100000)
```

## Programming Exercises

1. **Using Descriptive Procedures and ODS**

   a. Navigate to the SAS Help documentation and view the TABLES statement options for the FREQ procedure. Which option enables you to create a frequency plot? Use PROC FREQ to create one-way frequency tables for the variables **central_air** and **house_style** along with frequency plots. What percentage of homes in this sample have central air? What percent are only one story?

```
proc freq data=sp4r.ameshousing;
   tables central_air house_style / plots=freqplot;
run;
```

Selected PROC FREQ option:

PLOTS: use the FREQPLOT option to display a frequency plot (bar chart) of the corresponding frequency table.

| The FREQ Procedure | | | | |
| --- | --- | --- | --- | --- |
| Central_ Air | Frequency | Percent | Cumulative Frequency | Cumulative Percent |
| N | 42 | 14.00 | 42 | 14.00 |
| Y | 258 | 86.00 | 300 | 100.00 |

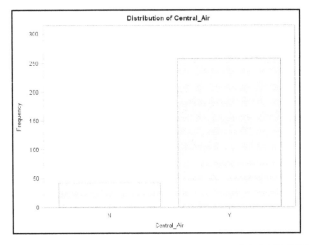

| House_ Style | Frequency | Percent | Cumulative Frequency | Cumulative Percent |
| --- | --- | --- | --- | --- |
| 1.5Fin | 28 | 9.33 | 28 | 9.33 |
| 1.5Unf | 4 | 1.33 | 32 | 10.67 |
| 1Story | 194 | 64.67 | 226 | 75.33 |
| 2.5Unf | 2 | 0.67 | 228 | 76.00 |
| 2Story | 38 | 12.67 | 266 | 88.67 |
| SFoyer | 13 | 4.33 | 279 | 93.00 |
| SLvl | 21 | 7.00 | 300 | 100.00 |

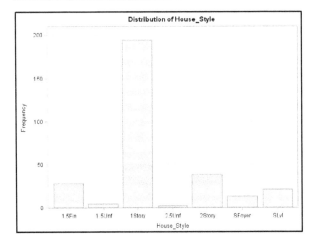

b.  The default PROC CORR output gives a table of simple statistics and correlation coefficients. Use ODS SELECT to print only the correlation coefficients for the variables **saleprice**, **garage_area**, **basement_area**, and **gr_liv_area**. (Hint: It might be easiest to use the ODS TRACE statement to learn the table name instead of going to the documentation page.) Is there a statistically significant correlation between **saleprice** and each of the other variables?

```
ods select pearsoncorr;
proc corr data=sp4r.ameshousing;
    var saleprice garage_area basement_area gr_liv_area;
run;
```

```
                            The CORR Procedure

                  Pearson Correlation Coefficients, N = 300
                       Prob > |r| under H0: Rho=0

                           Sale       Garage_      Basement_       Gr_Liv_
                          Price         Area           Area          Area
         SalePrice      1.00000       0.57892        0.08956       0.65046
                                       <.0001         <.0001        <.0001


         Garage_Area    0.57892       1.00000        0.35630       0.33283
                         <.0001                       <.0001        <.0001


         Basement_Area  0.08956       0.35630        1.00000       0.43985
                         <.0001        <.0001                       <.0001


         Gr_Liv_Area    0.65046       0.33283        0.43985       1.00000
                         <.0001        <.0001         <.0001
```

c.   Use PROC MEANS to print the 10th percentile, median, and 90th percentile for the variables **saleprice** and **gr_liv_area**. In addition, use the CLASS statement to separate the summary statistics by the **yr_sold** variable. Finally, save the output using ODS OUTPUT and name the table **summary_table**. Print the table to ensure it is saved. Which year had the highest median sale price?

```
ods output summary=summary_table;
proc means data=sp4r.ameshousing p10 median p90;
    var saleprice gr_liv_area;
    class yr_sold;
run;

proc print data=summary_table;
run;
```

Selected PROC MEANS statement:

CLASS specifies the variables whose values define the subgroup combinations for the analysis. Class variables are numeric or character. Class variables can have continuous values, but they typically have a few discrete values that define levels of the variable.

```
                        VName_     SalePrice_   SalePrice_   SalePrice_
Obs     Yr_Sold   NObs  SalePrice      P10        Median         P90

 1        2006      55   SalePrice     93500       131000       169000
 2        2007      72   SalePrice     96500       128500       180500
 3        2008      62   SalePrice     87000       130250       181900
 4        2009      73   SalePrice     91300       144000       192000
 5        2010      38   SalePrice    100000       148875       192000


        VName_Gr_   Gr_Liv_Area_   Gr_Liv_Area_   Gr_Liv_Area_
Obs     Liv_Area        P10          Median           P90

 1      Gr_Liv_Area      864          1092            1368
 2      Gr_Liv_Area      864          1070            1435
 3      Gr_Liv_Area      864          1185            1430
 4      Gr_Liv_Area      800          1210            1450
 5      Gr_Liv_Area      848          1148.5          1395
```

d.   Use PROC UNIVARIATE to analyze the **gr_liv_area** variable and create both a histogram and a QQPlot. For the histogram, overlay a normal and density kernel estimate. Use the OUTPUT statement to create a new data table of percentiles called **gr_percs**. Instead of providing the PCTLPTS= option a list, use the following syntax: `PCTLPTS= 40 to 60 by 2`. Let the prefixes for the saved percentiles be **gr_**. Print the table to ensure that it is saved.

```
proc univariate data=sp4r.ameshousing;
    var gr_liv_area;
    histogram gr_liv_area / normal kernel;
    qqplot gr_liv_area / normal(mu=est sigma=est);
    output out=gr_percs pctlpts= 40 to 60 by 2
        pctlpre=gr_liv_area_;
    run;

proc print data=gr_percs;
run;
```

Selected PROC UNIVARIATE statements and options:

OUT specifies the name of the new SAS data table.

PCTLPTS specifies the percentiles to be calculated for the VAR statement variables.

PCTLPRE specifies one or more prefixes for the name of the variable to be created followed by the percentile listed in the PCTLPTS option.

VAR specifies numeric variables to analyze.

HISTOGRAM specifies the numeric variable that is used to create a histogram. Use the NORMAL and KERNEL option to overlay a normal density and kernel density estimate.

INSET specifies which statistics to include in the histogram plot. Use the POSITION= option to provide a location. Provide the option with a compass direction (NE = North East).

QQPLOT specifies numeric variables to create a Q-Q plot. Use the NORMAL option to add a line to the Q-Q plot. Use the MU= and SIGMA= options to specify the parameters of the distribution for which quantiles are compared.

```
                    The UNIVARIATE Procedure
                     Variable:  Gr_Liv_Area

                            Moments

N                      300     Sum Weights              300
Mean                1130.74    Sum Observations      339222
Std Deviation    232.649389    Variance           54125.7382
Skewness         -0.3905489    Kurtosis           -0.3328098
Uncorrected SS    399755480    Corrected SS       16183595.7
Coeff Variation  20.5749676    Std Error Mean     13.4320187

                   Basic Statistical Measures

          Location                    Variability

     Mean     1130.740    Std Deviation       232.64939
     Median   1135.000    Variance                54126
     Mode      864.000    Range                    1166
                          Interquartile Range  385.50000

                  Tests for Location: Mu0=0

     Test              -Statistic-      -----p Value------

     Student's t    t   64.18243    Pr > |t|     <.0001
     Sign           M       150     Pr >= |M|    <.0001
     Signed Rank    S     22575     Pr >= |S|    <.0001

                  Quantiles (Definition 5)

                  Level         Quantile

                  100% Max        1500.0
                  99%             1490.0
                  95%             1466.0
                  90%             1431.0
                  75% Q3          1337.5
```

```
                  50% Median      1135.0
                  25% Q1           952.0
                  10%              847.0
                  5%               768.0
                  1%               509.0
                  0% Min           334.0
```

```
                  Extreme Observations

          ----Lowest----        ----Highest---

          Value      Obs        Value      Obs

            334      190         1484      142
            438      100         1486       95
            498      294         1494      181
            520      145         1494      290
            599       70         1500      222
```

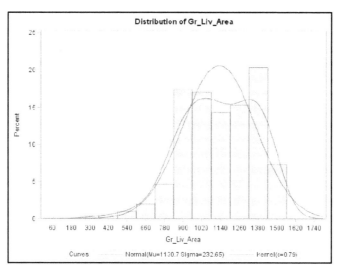

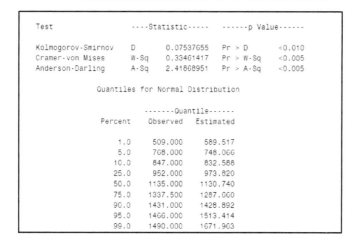

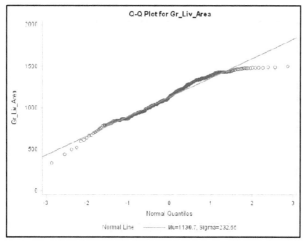

| Obs | gr_40 | gr_42 | gr_44 | gr_46 | gr_48 | gr_50 | gr_52 | gr_54 | gr_56 | gr_58 | gr_60 |
|-----|-------|-------|-------|-------|--------|-------|-------|--------|-------|-------|-------|
| 1 | 1063.5 | 1075.5 | 1087 | 1092 | 1109.5 | 1135 | 1151 | 1169.5 | 1191 | 1200 | 1218 |

2. **Creating and Using a Macro Variable for Unsupervised Scripting**

   a. Use the MEANS procedure to create a new data table with the median of the **SalePrice** variable.

   ```
   proc means data=sp4r.ameshousing;
       var saleprice;
       output out=sp4r.stats median=sp_med;
   run;
   ```

   b. Use PROC SQL to create a macro variable of the median **SalePrice** value.

   ```
   proc sql;
       select sp_med into :sp_med from sp4r.stats;
   quit;
   ```

   | sp_med |
   |--------|
   | 135000 |

   c. In the **AmesHousing** data set, create a new variable that is a value of *1* if the **SalePrice** is greater than the median and *0* otherwise. Use PROC FREQ to create a frequency table of the new variable.

   ```
   data sp4r.ameshousing;
       set sp4r.ameshousing;
       if saleprice > &sp_med then sp_bin = 1;
       else sp_bin = 0;
   run;

   proc freq data=sp4r.ameshousing;
       tables sp_bin;
   run;
   ```

   The FREQ Procedure

   | sp_bin | Frequency | Percent | Cumulative Frequency | Cumulative Percent |
   |--------|-----------|---------|----------------------|--------------------|
   | 0 | 153 | 51.00 | 153 | 51.00 |
   | 1 | 147 | 49.00 | 300 | 100.00 |

3. **Using the SYMPUTX Subroutine**

   a. The SYMPUTX subroutine enables you to create a macro variable inside a DATA step. Navigate to the online documentation for a complete description. Run the SAS code below (**SP4R05e03.sas**) and analyze both the code and log output. What does this code do?

   ```
   data _NULL_;
       x=-3;
       df=5;
       p=(1-probt(abs(x),df))*2;
       call symputx('sig_level',p);
   run;


   %put The significance level for the two-tailed t test is
       &sig_level;
   ```

   ```
   The significance level for the two-tailed t test is 0.0300992479
   ```

   This code uses a DATA _NULL_ step to create a macro variable for the significance level of a two-sided *t* test with five degrees of freedom and a test value of -3.

   Selected functions and subroutines:

   PROBT(x,df) returns the probability that an observation form a Student's distribution, with degrees of freedom **df**, is less than or equal to **x**.

   SYMPUTX assigns a value to a macro variable and removes both leading and trailing blanks.

b.  An alternative method to creating the macro variable in Exercise 2 is to use the SYMPUTX subroutine. Use a DATA _NULL_ step, a SET statement, and the SYMPUTX routine to create a macro variable for the median of the **saleprice** variable. Use the %PUT statement to ensure that the macro variable is created correctly.

```
proc means data=sp4r.ameshousing;
    var saleprice;
    output out=stats median=sp_med;
run;

data _null_;
    set stats;
    call symputx('med',sp_med);
run;


%put The median of the Sale Price variable is &med;
```

```
The median of the Sale Price variable is 135000
```

4.  **Creating a Macro to Generate Summary Statistics and Plots of Any Data Table**

a.  Open **SP4R05e04.sas**. Create the **mystats** macro. It should have a single positional parameter (**dt**) and four keyword parameters (**freq**=*no*, **means**=*no*, **opts**= , and **scatter**=*no*). Use the %IF, %THEN, and %END macro statements to validate the positional parameter. If no data table (**dt**) is supplied by the user, use %PUT to write the sentence "dt is a required argument" to the log and use the %RETURN statement to terminate the macro.

```
%macro mystats(dt,freq=no,corr=no,means=no,opts=,scatter=no);

%if &dt= %then %do;
    %put dt is a required argument;
    %return;
%end;
```

b.  Use PROC CONTENTS with the OUT= option to write the contents of the input data table (**dt**) to a new data table called **dtcontents**. Use PROC SQL to use the **Name** field from **dtcontents** to create two macro variables. Let **vars_cont** be the unique names of continuous variables in the data set separated by a space. Let **vars_cat** be the unique names of the categorical variables in the data set separated by a space.

```
proc contents data=&dt varnum out=dtcontents;
run;

proc sql;
    select distinct name into: vars_cont separated by ' '
        from dtcontents where type=1;
    select distinct NAME into: vars_cat separated by ' '
        from dtcontents where type=2;
quit;
```

c.  Use macro statements to generate a PROC FREQ step if the user supplied **freq**=*yes* when calling **mystats**. In this case, use PROC FREQ to create frequency tables for the categorical variables.

```
%if %upcase(&freq)=YES %then %do;
    proc freq data=&dt;
        tables &vars_cat;
    run;
%end;
```

d.  Use macro statements to generate a PROC MEANS step if the user supplies **means**=*yes*. In this case, specify the continuous variables in the VAR statement. In addition, use the **opts** parameter in the PROC MEANS statement to easily change the descriptive statistics.

```
%if %upcase(&means)=YES %then %do;
    proc means data=&dt &opts;
        var &vars_cont;
    run;
%end;
```

e. Use macro statements to set a condition if the user supplies **scatter**=*yes*. In this case, use PROC SGSCATTER to create a scatter plot matrix of the continuous variables. End the creation of the macro with %MEND.

```
%if %upcase(&scatter)=YES %then %do;
    proc sgscatter data=&dt;
        matrix &vars_cont;
    run;
%end;
%mend;
```

f. Call the **mystats** macro to create frequency tables for the **cars** data set.

```
%mystats(sp4r.cars,freq=yes)
```

The FREQ Procedure

| Drive Train | Frequency | Percent | Cumulative Frequency | Cumulative Percent |
|---|---|---|---|---|
| All | 92 | 21.50 | 92 | 21.50 |
| Front | 226 | 52.80 | 318 | 74.30 |
| Rear | 110 | 25.70 | 428 | 100.00 |

| Make | Frequency | Percent | Cumulative Frequency | Cumulative Percent |
|---|---|---|---|---|
| Acura | 7 | 1.64 | 7 | 1.64 |
| Audi | 19 | 4.44 | 26 | 6.07 |
| BMW | 20 | 4.67 | 46 | 10.75 |
| Buick | 9 | 2.10 | 55 | 12.85 |
| Cadillac | 8 | 1.87 | 63 | 14.72 |
| Chevrolet | 27 | 6.31 | 90 | 21.03 |
| Chrysler | 15 | 3.50 | 105 | 24.53 |
| Dodge | 13 | 3.04 | 118 | 27.57 |
| Ford | 23 | 5.37 | 141 | 32.94 |
| GMC | 8 | 1.87 | 149 | 34.81 |
| Honda | 17 | 3.97 | 166 | 38.79 |

| | Frequency | Percent | Cumulative Frequency | Cumulative Percent |
|---|---|---|---|---|
| Hummer | 1 | 0.23 | 167 | 39.02 |
| Hyundai | 12 | 2.80 | 179 | 41.82 |
| Infiniti | 8 | 1.87 | 187 | 43.69 |
| Isuzu | 2 | 0.47 | 189 | 44.16 |
| Jaguar | 12 | 2.80 | 201 | 46.96 |
| Jeep | 3 | 0.70 | 204 | 47.66 |
| Kia | 11 | 2.57 | 215 | 50.23 |
| Land Rover | 3 | 0.70 | 218 | 50.93 |
| Lexus | 11 | 2.57 | 229 | 53.50 |
| Lincoln | 9 | 2.10 | 238 | 55.61 |
| MINI | 2 | 0.47 | 240 | 56.07 |
| Mazda | 11 | 2.57 | 251 | 58.64 |
| Mercedes-Benz | 26 | 6.07 | 277 | 64.72 |
| Mercury | 9 | 2.10 | 286 | 66.82 |
| Mitsubishi | 13 | 3.04 | 299 | 69.86 |
| Nissan | 17 | 3.97 | 316 | 73.83 |
| Oldsmobile | 3 | 0.70 | 319 | 74.53 |
| Pontiac | 11 | 2.57 | 330 | 77.10 |
| Porsche | 7 | 1.64 | 337 | 78.74 |
| Saab | 7 | 1.64 | 344 | 80.37 |
| Saturn | 8 | 1.87 | 352 | 82.24 |
| Scion | 2 | 0.47 | 354 | 82.71 |
| Subaru | 11 | 2.57 | 365 | 85.28 |
| Suzuki | 8 | 1.87 | 373 | 87.15 |
| Toyota | 28 | 6.54 | 401 | 93.69 |
| Volkswagen | 15 | 3.50 | 416 | 97.20 |
| Volvo | 12 | 2.80 | 428 | 100.00 |

Partial Model Table

The FREQ Procedure

| Model | Frequency | Percent | Cumulative Frequency | Cumulative Percent |
|---|---|---|---|---|
| 3.5 RL 4dr | 1 | 0.23 | 1 | 0.23 |
| 3.5 RL w/Navigation 4dr | 1 | 0.23 | 2 | 0.47 |
| 300M 4dr | 1 | 0.23 | 3 | 0.70 |
| 300M Special Edition 4dr | 1 | 0.23 | 4 | 0.93 |
| 325Ci 2dr | 1 | 0.23 | 5 | 1.17 |
| 325Ci convertible 2dr | 1 | 0.23 | 6 | 1.40 |

| Origin | Frequency | Percent | Cumulative Frequency | Cumulative Percent |
|---|---|---|---|---|
| Asia | 158 | 36.92 | 158 | 36.92 |
| Europe | 123 | 28.74 | 281 | 65.65 |
| USA | 147 | 34.35 | 428 | 100.00 |

| Type | Frequency | Percent | Cumulative Frequency | Cumulative Percent |
|---|---|---|---|---|
| Hybrid | 3 | 0.70 | 3 | 0.70 |
| SUV | 60 | 14.02 | 63 | 14.72 |
| Sedan | 262 | 61.21 | 325 | 75.93 |
| Sports | 49 | 11.45 | 374 | 87.38 |
| Truck | 24 | 5.61 | 398 | 92.99 |
| Wagon | 30 | 7.01 | 428 | 100.00 |

g. Call the **mystats** macro to create the means output with `opts=mean median maxdec=2`. Generate a scatter plot matrix for the continuous variables.

```
%mystats(sp4r.cars,means=yes,opts=mean median
    maxdec=2,scatter=yes)
```

The MEANS Procedure

| Variable | Label | Mean | Median |
|---|---|---|---|
| Cylinders | | 5.81 | 6.00 |
| EngineSize | Engine Size (L) | 3.20 | 3.00 |
| Horsepower | | 215.89 | 210.00 |
| Invoice | | 30014.70 | 25294.50 |
| Length | Length (IN) | 186.36 | 187.00 |
| MPG_City | MPG (City) | 20.06 | 19.00 |
| MPG_Highway | MPG (Highway) | 26.84 | 26.00 |
| MSRP | | 32774.86 | 27635.00 |
| Weight | Weight (LBS) | 3577.95 | 3474.50 |
| Wheelbase | Wheelbase (IN) | 108.15 | 107.00 |

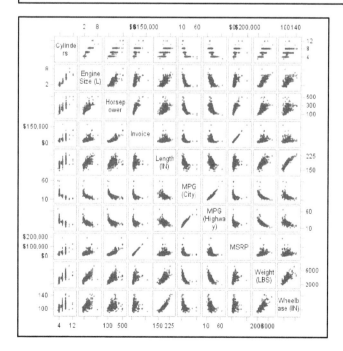

5. **Creating a Macro for Iterative Processing**

Import a series of Excel workbook sheets into corresponding SAS data sets. The **amesbyyear** Excel workbook contains five separate sheets. Each sheet holds only the information for homes sold in a specific year. Each sheet is named according to the year (2006, 2007, 2008, 2009, 2010). The data begins on row 2, and row 1 contains all the variable names.

a.  Create a macro to iteratively call PROC IMPORT to read in each sheet of the **amesbyyear** spreadsheet. Call the macro **myimport** and give it two positional parameters (**firstyear**, **lastyear**). Let each new data set (one for each sheet) be named **year20##** where ## refers to each specific year.

> Remember that the iteration index value can be referenced as a macro variable.

```
%macro myimport(firstyear,lastyear);
    %do i=&firstyear %to &lastyear;
        proc import datafile = "&path\amesbyyear.xlsx"
            out = sp4r.year&i
            dbms = xlsx REPLACE;
            getnames = yes;
            sheet = "&i";
            datarow = 2;
        run;
    %end;
%mend;
```

b.  Call **myimport** to read in each sheet of the Excel file.

```
options mprint;
%myimport(2006,2010)
```

```
5078  options mprint;
5079  %myimport(2006,2010)
MPRINT(MYIMPORT):   proc import out = year2006 datafile =
"C:\Users\jobake\Desktop\sp4rtest\amesbyyear.xlsx" dbms = xlsx REPLACE;
MPRINT(MYIMPORT):   RXLX;
MPRINT(MYIMPORT):   getnames = yes;
MPRINT(MYIMPORT):   sheet = "2006";
MPRINT(MYIMPORT):   datarow = 2;
MPRINT(MYIMPORT):   run;

MPRINT(MYIMPORT):   proc import out = year2007 datafile =
"C:\Users\jobake\Desktop\sp4rtest\amesbyyear.xlsx" dbms = xlsx REPLACE;
MPRINT(MYIMPORT):   RXLX;
MPRINT(MYIMPORT):   getnames = yes;
MPRINT(MYIMPORT):   sheet = "2007";
MPRINT(MYIMPORT):   datarow = 2;
MPRINT(MYIMPORT):   run;

MPRINT(MYIMPORT):   proc import out = year2008 datafile =
"C:\Users\jobake\Desktop\sp4rtest\amesbyyear.xlsx" dbms = xlsx REPLACE;
MPRINT(MYIMPORT):   RXLX;
MPRINT(MYIMPORT):   getnames = yes;
MPRINT(MYIMPORT):   sheet = "2008";
MPRINT(MYIMPORT):   datarow = 2;
MPRINT(MYIMPORT):   run;
```

```
MPRINT(MYIMPORT):   proc import out = year2009 datafile =
"C:\Users\jobake\Desktop\sp4rtest\amesbyyear.xlsx" dbms = xlsx REPLACE;
MPRINT(MYIMPORT):   RXLX;
MPRINT(MYIMPORT):   getnames = yes;
MPRINT(MYIMPORT):   sheet = "2009";
MPRINT(MYIMPORT):   datarow = 2;
MPRINT(MYIMPORT):   run;

MPRINT(MYIMPORT):   proc import out = year2010 datafile =
"C:\Users\jobake\Desktop\sp4rtest\amesbyyear.xlsx" dbms = xlsx REPLACE;
MPRINT(MYIMPORT):   RXLX;
MPRINT(MYIMPORT):   getnames = yes;
MPRINT(MYIMPORT):   sheet = "2010";
MPRINT(MYIMPORT):   datarow = 2;
MPRINT(MYIMPORT):   run;
```

c.  Check the **SP4R** library to ensure that all five data sets are created.

# Chapter 6: Analyzing the Data via Inferential Procedures

## Introduction

In the previous chapters, you learned how to import your data into SAS, alter the data to meet your specifications, and create graphics and summary statistics to get a feel for the data. You are now ready to begin creating some statistical models. We will practice using inferential procedures in SAS with a whole slew of linear, generalized linear, and mixed models.

SAS modeling procedure syntax is very consistent. After you master the syntax required to create these models, you will have no problem extending your own statistical knowledge to time series, Bayesian, or survival procedures, to name a few.

## Linear Models

In this section, we will create lots of different linear models including a multiple linear regression, analysis of variance, analysis of covariance, and finally, we will get into a little bit of effect selection. We will hypothesize a linear model, use an appropriate PROC step to create the linear model and generate both tables and statistical graphics, and then save the important model information with the OUTPUT statement that we have learned before.

For linear models, we would use the LM function in R for regression, polynomial regression, ANOVA, and so on, as shown in Figure 6.1. We just tack on the AS.FACTOR function to indicate a classification variable, and an analysis of covariance when we have both classification variables and continuous variables. You will learn how to reproduce the ANOVA, SUMMARY, and PLOT functions applied to your model object.

**Figure 6.1: R Script**

```
     Source on Save    Q  / ▾             →Run   ⇥   →Source
#Regression
mylm ← lm(SalePrice ~ Gr_Liv_Area + Age_Sold)
mylm; summary(mylm); anova(mylm)
par(mfrow=c(2,2)); plot(mylm)

#Polynomial
x2 = x^2; x3 = x^3; x4 = x^4; x5 = x^5
mylm ← lm(y ~ x + x2 + x3 + x4 + x5)
mylm; summary(mylm); anova(mylm)
par(mfrow=c(2,2)); plot(mylm)

#ANOVA
mylm ← lm(SalePrice ~ as.factor(Heating_QC))
mylm; anova(mylm); summary(mylm)
par(mfrow=c(2,2)); plot(mylm)

#ANCOVA
mylm ← lm(SalePrice ~ as.factor(Heating_QC) + Gr_Liv_Area
        + as.factor(Heating_QC)*Gr_Liv_Area)
mylm; anova(mylm); summary(mylm)
par(mfrow=c(2,2))
plot(mylm)
```

## PROC REG

PROC REG can be used to create a simple linear regression or multiple linear regression model. In PROC REG, we are only going to specify continuous predictors. If you wanted to dummy-code your own variable to create classification variables, you could do that, but we will see how to create a classification variable explicitly in SAS using PROC GLM a little bit later.

To specify your model, we will simply use the MODEL statement as shown in the following syntax:

**PROC REG DATA=***data-set-name*;
   **MODEL** *dependent-variable = regressors </ options>*;
**RUN; QUIT;**

> **Tip**: Variables specified in the MODEL statement must be numeric variables.

### Simple Linear Regression

In Program 6.1, we are creating a simple linear regression model using the ameshousing data set. The dependent variable is on the left (saleprice), and we set that equal to all the regressors in the model. In this case, there is only one: the gr_liv_area, and you do not need to use your plus symbols to add in predictors. You just simply list them after the equal sign.

**Program 6.1: PROC REG**

```
proc reg data=ameshousing;
    model saleprice = gr_liv_area;
run;quit;
```

**Output 6.1: Results of Program 6.1**

| Analysis of Variance | | | | | |
|---|---|---|---|---|---|
| Source | DF | Sum of Squares | Mean Square | F Value | Pr > F |
| Model | 1 | 1.790671E11 | 1.790671E11 | 218.56 | < .0001 |
| Error | 298 | 2.441564E11 | 819316790 | | |
| Corrected Total | 299 | 4.232235E11 | | | |

| Root MSE | | 28624 | R-Square | 0 4231 |
| Dependent Mean | | 137525 | Adj R-Sq | 0 4212 |
| Coeff Var | | 20 81348 | | |

**Parameter Estimates**

| Variable | DF | Parameter Estimate | Standard Error | t Value | Pr > \|t\| |
| --- | --- | --- | --- | --- | --- |
| Intercept | 1 | 18583 | 8213 43837 | 2 26 | 0 0244 |
| Gr_Liv_Area | 1 | 105 18902 | 7 11522 | 14 78 | < 0001 |

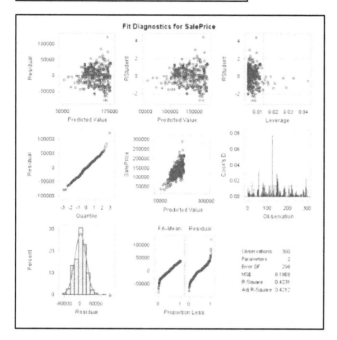

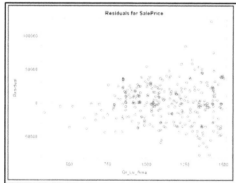

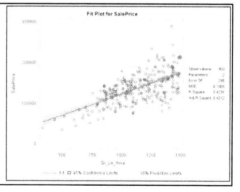

As shown in Output 6.1, by default we get similar output to the SUMMARY and ANOVA functions applied to the model object (for example, when you get the analysis of variance table), and also our parameter estimates with standard errors, t values, and *p*-values. We also get a little bit of other information like the root mean square error, R square, and so on. By default, PROC REG will give you a diagnostics panel, and a lot of this information is the same as plotting the model object in R. For example, we get the Residual by Predicted plot, R studentized Residuals by the Predicted Values, R studentized Residuals by Leverage, and so on.

> **Tip:** Use the PLOTS(UNPACK) option in the PROC REG statement to plot the default output individually, without a panel.

The one output that you do not get from plotting the model object in R is the Cook's Distance plot by Observation, but this is just a measure of how predicted scores change when observations are removed from the model, so it is trying to identify outliers. You can see in the Fit Diagnostics in Output 6.1, at observation 125, the Cook's Distance is very large, indicating this is a possible outlier.

Also, by default, you will get the Residual by the Predictor Value graphic, so for every regressor that you have in your model, it will create a single Residual by Regressor plot. And if you are doing a simple linear regression model, SAS will go ahead and give you the simple linear regression plot. It will tack on that line of best fit, your confidence limits, and prediction limits, by default.

## Polynomial Regression

To do polynomial regression in SAS, we have to begin the same way as we would in R. Specifically, we had to add those regressors to our existing SAS data set. In Program 6.2, you can see we are adding x squared, x cubed, all the way through x to the fifth power. We are adding those polynomial regressors to our data set, and then we can use them in PROC REG.

**Program 6.2: Preparation for Polynomial Regression**

```
data mydata;
    set mydata;
    x2 = x**2; x3 = x**3; x4 = x**4; x5 = x**5;
run;
```

> **Tip**: Recall that SAS does not use the ^ symbol for exponentiation. It uses the double star symbol.

## PROC PLM

To reproduce the PREDICT function in R, we can use the PLM procedure to score new SAS data sets. We begin the same way as we would in R. Specifically, in R, we create a model object. In SAS, we are going to store the model with the STORE statement inside the procedure using the following syntax:

**STORE** *item-store-name*;

In Program 6.3, we are running PROC REG with whatever MODEL statement you want to use, and storing the model with the STORE statement under the mymod name. Once we save the model, then we can pass it to the PLM procedure like we would pass the model object to the PREDICT function.

**Program 6.3: Save the Model with the STORE Statement**

```
proc reg data=ameshousing;
    ...
    store mymod;
run;
```

The STORE statement requests that the procedure save the context and results of the statistical analysis. The resulting item store has a binary file format that cannot be modified. The contents of the item store can be processed with the PLM procedure.

In the R Script in Figure 6.1, we passed the model object to the PREDICT function, and then the new data set we want to score. In SAS, we are going to pass the model to the PLM procedure using the RESTORE= option with the following syntax:

**PROC PLM RESTORE=***item-store-specification*;
    **SCORE DATA=***new-data-set*
          **OUT =***predicted-data-set <keywords>*;
**RUN;**

In Program 6.4, we restore mymod, which we specified in the STORE statement of the SAS procedure PROC REG in Program 6.3. We use the SCORE statement, and specify the DATA= option to tell SAS the new SAS data set we are scoring—in this case, newdata. SAS is going to use the model specified in the RESTORE option to predict values for the new data set. You can also use the OUT= option to save the new scored values. We are calling the new data set pred, for predicted.

**Program 6.4: PROC PLM**

```
proc plm restore=mymod;
    score data=newdata out=pred;
run;
```

You can also pass a bunch of other keywords to the PROC PLM SCORE statement to generate other output. For example, you can generate predicted values, standard errors, residuals, confidence limits, and also prediction limits as shown in Table 6.1.

**Table 6.1: SCORE Statement Keywords**

| Keyword | Description |
| --- | --- |
| PREDICTED | Linear predictor |
| STDERR | Standard Error |
| RESIDUAL | Residual |
| LCLM | Lower confidence limit |
| UCLM | Upper confidence limit |
| LCL | Lower prediction limit |
| UCL | Upper prediction limit |

**Tip**: If you want to change from an alpha level of 0.05, just use the ALPHA= option for your limits.

The STORE statement to save your model is supported by most of the SAS/STAT procedures. In this book, we are going to use it in PROC REG, GLM, GLMSELECT, LOGISTIC, GENMOD, and MIXED. There are a few procedures where you can score data right in the procedure where you are creating your model. Specifically, you can use the SCORE statement in PROC GLMSELECT and PROC LOGISTIC to bypass the use of PROC PLM. In this book we will always use the STORE statement in the modeling procedure, and then pass that to PROC PLM to score new data set. This is very similar to using the PREDICT function in R, but you should be aware of the SCORE statement in both the GLMSELECT and LOGISTIC procedures.

## PROC GLM

In this section, we move on from PROC REG to PROC GLM, which stands for the general linear model. In this case, we are going to perform an ANOVA and also an analysis of covariance. So we are moving away from PROC REG with just continuous variables and now we can use classification variables in PROC GLM as shown in the following syntax:

**PROC GLM DATA=***data-table-name*;
   **CLASS** *variables <options>*;
   **MODEL** *dependent-variable = independent-variables </options>*;
**RUN;**

In Program 6.5, we continue working with the ameshousing data set. To do an analysis of variance, choose the heating_qc (for quality control) in that data set. This variable has four levels: Excellent, Good, Average, and Fair. To tell SAS explicitly that it is a classification variable, use the CLASS statement and specify the variable heating_qc.

**Program 6.5: PROC GLM**

```
proc glm data=ameshousing;
    class heating_qc (ref='Fa');  ❶
    model saleprice = heating_qc / solution;  ❷
run; quit;
```

❶  The CLASS statement is identical to the AS.FACTOR function in R, so it is going to create a column in the design matrix for each classification level. As an option in parentheses, we specify the reference level. In this case, we set it equal to Fa for fair. That is case sensitive and it is as appears in the data set.

❷  Next, we use the MODEL statement the same way as in PROC REG. Set saleprice equal to the classification variable, heating_qc.

---

**Tip:** The CLASS statement in PROC GLM creates columns in the design matrix for each classification variable. The number of columns is the same as the number of levels in the CLASS variable. The value of each design column is either 0 or 1 across all observations.

---

**Output 6.5: Results of Program 6.5**

| Source | DF | Sum of Squares | Mean Square | F Value | Pr > F |
|---|---|---|---|---|---|
| Model | 3 | 66835556221 | 22278518740 | 18.50 | <.0001 |
| Error | 296 | 356387963289 | 1204013389.5 | | |
| Corrected Total | 299 | 423223519511 | | | |

| R-Square | Coeff Var | Root MSE | SalePrice Mean |
|---|---|---|---|
| 0.157920 | 25.23100 | 34698.90 | 137524.9 |

| Source | DF | Type I SS | Mean Square | F Value | Pr > F |
|---|---|---|---|---|---|
| Heating_QC | 3 | 66835556221 | 22278518740 | 18.50 | <.0001 |

| Source | DF | Type III SS | Mean Square | F Value | Pr > F |
|---|---|---|---|---|---|
| Heating_QC | 3 | 66835556221 | 22278518740 | 18.50 | <.0001 |

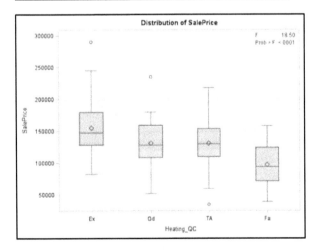

| Parameter | Estimate | | Standard Error | t Value | Pr > |t| |
|---|---|---|---|---|---|
| Intercept | 97118.75000 | B | 8674.724021 | 11.20 | <.0001 |
| Heating_QC Ex | 57800.43692 | B | 9300.714942 | 6.21 | <.0001 |
| Heating_QC Gd | 33725.33621 | B | 9798.453367 | 3.44 | 0.0007 |
| Heating_QC TA | 33454.77941 | B | 9239.512780 | 3.62 | 0.0003 |
| Heating_QC Fa | 0.00000 | B | | | |

By default, in Output 6.5 we get the analysis of variance table, which has an overall significant F test. We also get the R square, coefficient of variation, root mean square error, and the mean sale price. We also get the Type 1 and Type 3 sums of squares, which of course, when we only have one variable, are going to be identical.

One of the great things about SAS is that it is always giving you relevant statistical graphics. SAS knows we are doing a one-way analysis of variance, so in this case, it outputs a side-by-side box plot. For Excellent, it appears that the sale price on average is greater than Good, Average, and Fair. It appears that Good and Average are quite similar. And of course, the sale price for the Fair heating_qc (the lowest level) is associated with the lowest sale prices.

As a best practice, use the SOLUTION option in the MODEL statement to print the parameter estimates table. It displays the intercept, four levels, estimate, standard error, t value, and *p*-value. Notice the column in the middle that has the letter B In each element. That simply means that those terms are not uniquely estimable and there are no linear combinations of predictors to estimate those parameters individually.

## MEANS Statement

There are lots of different statements that can be used in PROC GLM, and going forward in this book, they will be quite consistent. Let's use the MEANS statement to specify our classification variables (in this case, heating_qc) using the following syntax:

**MEANS** *class-variable* < / HOVTEST=*test-name* >;

Using the MEANS statement in Program 6.6 gives us the default table shown in Output 6.6.

**Program 6.6: MEANS Statement**
```
proc glm data=ameshousing;
   ...
   means heating_qc / hovtest=bf;
run;quit;
```

**Output 6.6: Partial Results of Program 6.6**

| Level of Heating_QC | N | SalePrice Mean | Std Dev |
|---|---|---|---|
| Ex | 107 | 154919.187 | 36822.8795 |
| Gd | 58 | 130844.086 | 34912.5027 |
| TA | 119 | 130573.529 | 32177.4508 |
| Fa | 16 | 97118.750 | 37423.5437 |

Output 6.6 shows us the number of observations in each level (for example, Excellent has 107 observations), and it also gives me the mean and standard deviation. Another reason to use the MEAN statement is that you can use the HOVTEST option, the homogeneity of variance test. To test the assumption of equal variances, we have four options here as shown in Table 6.2.

**Table 6.2: HOVTEST Options**

| HOVTEST= | Homogeneity of Variance Test |
|----------|------------------------------|
| BARTLETT | Bartlett's Test |
| BF | Brown and Forsythe's Test |
| LEVENE | Levene's Test |
| OBRIEN | O'Brien's Test |

Check out the SAS documentation to see which option you might want to use.

## LSMEANS Statement

Another statement that can be used in PROC GLM is the LSMEANS statement, which stands for the least square means. Use the statement to add in the classification variables that you want to find the least square means for, as shown in the following syntax:

**LSMEANS** *class-variable < / options>*;

As an option, you can use the ADJUST= option to request multiple simultaneous comparisons. We can use the Tukey, Bonferroni, Dunnett, or Scheffe adjustments as shown in Table 6.3.

**Table 6.3: ADJUST= Options**

| ADJUST= | Homogeneity of Variance Test | Description |
|---------|------------------------------|-------------|
| TUKEY | Tukey Adjustment | Tukey is probably the test most users are familiar with. It tends to be the most powerful in most cases. |
| BON | Bonferroni Adjustment | This adjustment specifies an overall alpha and then that alpha is divvied up for each comparison. |
| DUNNET | Dunnett Adjustment | Dunnet is most frequently used when comparing everything to a control group. For example, if you are testing three drugs against a control, use the Dunnett adjustment because you would actually only be testing three comparisons in that case. |
| SCHEFFE | Scheffé Adjustment | The Scheffé adjustment controls for all possible comparisons. This is useful if you engage in data snooping. |

Also, by default, when you use the LSMEANS statement, of course, you get the least square mean for saleprice for each level of the classification variable, and you also get the comparison. In Program 6.7 and Output 6.7, we are comparing group 1 to group 2, and it has a *p*-value of 0.002 for the hypothesis test, which indicates the Excellent heating quality and Good heating quality are significantly different. On the other hand, comparing levels 2 to 3, comparing Good to Average, we can see that the *p*-value is definitely not less than 0.05, so these are not significantly different from each other.

**Program 6.7: LSMEANS Statement**

```
proc glm data=ameshousing;
    ...
    lsmeans heating_qc / adjust=tukey;
run;quit;
```

**Output 6.7: Results of Program 6.7**

| Heating_QC | SalePrice LSMEAN | LSMEAN Number |
|---|---|---|
| Ex | 154919.187 | 1 |
| Gd | 130844.086 | 2 |
| TA | 130573.529 | 3 |
| Fa | 97118.750 | 4 |

| Least Squares Means for effect Heating_QC Pr > \|t\| for H0: LSMean(i)=LSMean(j) Dependent Variable: SalePrice | | | | |
|---|---|---|---|---|
| i/j | 1 | 2 | 3 | 4 |
| 1 | | 0.0002 | < .0001 | < .0001 |
| 2 | 0.0002 | | 1.0000 | 0.0037 |
| 3 | < .0001 | 1.0000 | | 0.0020 |
| 4 | < .0001 | 0.0037 | 0.0020 | |

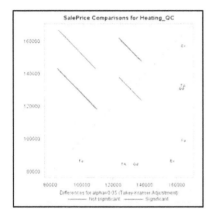

In Output 6.7, you can also see the default graphic, which has the same information as the comparison table. For example, Fair is significantly different from Average, Good, and Excellent, and we see that Average and Good are not significantly different.

## ESTIMATE Statement

Previously we talked about using PROC PLM to score new data sets. But what if you want to test a linear function of the parameters or a linear combination? In R, you could multiply the coefficients beta hat by a vector of coefficients L. That would give you your linear combination. In SAS, if you want to test main effects or simply estimate one single home price, you could do that directly in the ESTIMATE statement of the procedure. We will specify the vector L in the ESTIMATE statement using the following syntax:

**ESTIMATE** '*estimate-name*' *class-variable*
*linear-combination < / options>*;

This method is not for scoring entire data sets. The ESTIMATE statement only enables you to estimate linear functions of the parameters by creating the L matrix. The linear function is checked for estimability. The estimate of $L\beta$, where $\beta = (X'X)^{-}X'Y$ is displayed along with its associated standard error,

$$\sqrt{L(X'X)^{-}L's^2}$$ , and t test.

Let's look at an example. We want to test the linear combination mu1 equal to mu2, so we run PROC GLM with the appropriate statements as shown in Program 6.8.

**Program 6.8: ESTIMATE Statement**

```
proc glm data=ameshousing;
    ...  ❶
    estimate 'mu1 vs the rest'
        heating_qc 3 -1 -1 -1 / divisor=3;  ❷
run;quit;
```

❶  Here we are leaving out the MODEL statement just for space.

❷  In the ESTIMATE statement, we are going to test the main effects for mu1 equal to mu2. So first, we name the estimate. In quotation marks, specify mu1 minus mu2, and then pass it the classification variable, heating_qc. Then specify the coefficients for the L vector. We want a coefficient 1 for Excellent and -1 for Good; the rest all set as 0. If we omit the zeros, it would simply set all the remaining coefficients to zero where necessary.

Running Program 6.8 produces the table shown in Output 6.8.

**Output 6.8: Results of Program 6.8**

| Parameter | Estimate | Standard Error | t Value | Pr > \|t\| |
|---|---|---|---|---|
| mu1-mu2 | 24075.1007 | 5657.85411 | 4.26 | <.0001 |

In Output 6.8, we get an estimate of about $24,000. It appears that the sale price for homes with the Excellent heating condition are about $24,000 greater, on average, than homes with the Good heating condition. We also get the standard error, t value, and *p*-value. Here the *p*-value indicates that the main effect difference is statistically significant.

Let's look at another example testing the linear combination for $\widehat{\mu}_1 - \frac{\widehat{\mu}_2}{3} - \frac{\widehat{\mu}_3}{3} - \frac{\widehat{\mu}_4}{3}$. In Program 6.9, we have coefficients of minus a third for each of the other three levels, And in the ESTIMATE statement, we will specify the integer values: 3 minus 1 minus 1 minus 1. As an option, we will give it the divisor equal to 3. This is simply going to divide each one of the coefficients by 3 and produce the appropriate fractions.

**Program 6.9: ESTIMATE Statement for Linear Combination**

```
proc glm data=ameshousing;
    ...
    estimate 'mu1 vs the rest'
        heating_qc 3 -1 -1 -1 / divisor=3;
run;quit;
```

**Output 6.9: Results of Program 6.9**

| Parameter | Estimate | Standard Error | t Value | Pr > \|t\| |
|---|---|---|---|---|
| mu1 vs the rest | 35407.0650 | 4800.45834 | 7.38 | <.0001 |

In Output 6.9, we get an estimate of about $35,000, standard error, t value, and a significant *p*-value.

As a best practice, it is a good idea to use the E option in the ESTIMATE statement. That option will print your L vector to make sure you specify the coefficients correctly. In Program 6.10, we have an intercept with a coefficient of 0. Excellent has a coefficient of 1, And of course, the rest have coefficients of -1/3. Output 6.10 will be printed to the results page when you use the E option.

**Program 6.10: E Option in ESTIMATE Statement**

```
proc glm data=ameshousing;
    ...
    estimate 'mu1 vs the rest'
        heating_qc 3 -1 -1 -1 / e divisor=3;
run;quit;
```

**Output 6.10: Partial Results of Program 6.10**

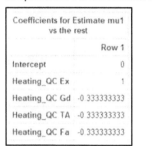

| Coefficients for Estimate mu1 vs the rest | |
|---|---|
| | Row 1 |
| Intercept | 0 |
| Heating_QC Ex | 1 |
| Heating_QC Gd | -0.333333333 |
| Heating_QC TA | -0.333333333 |
| Heating_QC Fa | -0.333333333 |

> Tip: The E option is useful when you confirm the ordering of parameters for specifying *L*.

So far, we have been talking about analysis of variance with just a single classification variable. In PROC GLM, we can add in continuous variables to an analysis of covariance such as the following ANCOVA model:

$Y_{ij} = \mu + \alpha_i + \beta_i X_{ij} + \theta_i X_{ij} + \varepsilon_{ij}$ . So, we can add in the predictor $X_{ij}$. We still have the classification

variable represented by alpha. Now we can estimate an overall slope and the slope adjustment for each level, but everything is going to be very consistent in PROC GLM. We are still going to use the CLASS, MODEL, LSMEANS, ESTIMATE, and OUTPUT statements.

## PROC GLMSELECT

To finish up this section on linear models, let's talk about stepwise model selection. Imagine we have lots and lots of different predictors. We want to run those predictors through some type of procedure and get back a more parsimonious model. To do so, we are going to use PROC GLMSELECT to perform effect selection. This is only for general linear models framework, but fitting the model is exactly the same as the procedures that we discussed earlier in this section. We are going to use the same CLASS and MODEL statements. The only difference here is we are going to specify different options to do the effect selection.

PROC GLMSELECT, in general, combines the features of PROC GLM and PROC REG, so you can do all your general linear models, all your multiple linear regression, ANOVA, analysis of covariance right in PROC GLMSELECT using the following syntax:

**PROC GLMSELECT DATA=**=*data-table-name*;
   **CLASS** *categorical-variables*;
   **MODEL** *dependent-variable = model-effects / options*;
**RUN;**

On the other hand, you might prefer to use the three separate procedures that we have talked about so far in this section because they tend to give you different graphical output. For example, in PROC GLM, when it knows you are doing a one-way analysis of variance, it automatically gives you a side-by-side box plot. That might not be the case when using in PROC GLMSELECT.

### SELECTION= Option

If you want to do multiple linear aggression, ANOVA, ANCOVA, in PROC GLMSELECT, choose the SELECTION= option to specify a selection method and specify it as NONE. So, no model selection; just simply fit the model.

On the other hand, if you want to do effect selection in PROC GLMSELECT, we can use the following methods shown in Table 6.4.

Table 6.4: SELECTION= Options

| SELECTION= | Description |
|---|---|
| NONE | No model selection. |
| FORWARD | Forward selection. The model starts with no effects and iteratively adds in effects according to some criteria. |
| BACKWARD | Backward selection. The model starts with all effects in the model already and deletes effects according to some criteria. |
| STEPWISE | Stepwise regression; similar to the FORWARD method except effects in the model do not necessarily stay in the model. That is not the case in FORWARD selection. In FORWARD selection, if it is in the model, it stays in the model. |
| LAR | Least angle regression; similar to the FORWARD method except parameter estimates are shrunk. |
| LASSO | Specifies the LASSO method, which adds and deletes parameters based on a version of ordinary least squares where the sum of the absolute regression coefficients is constrained. |
| ELASTICNET | An extension of LASSO. Both the sum of the absolute regression coefficients and the sum of the squared regression coefficients are constrained. |
| GROUPLASSO | A variant of LASSO. Based on a version of ordinary least squares in which the sum of the Euclidean norms, a group of regression coefficients is constrained. |

**Tip**: If the SELECTION= option is omitted, the default is SELECTION=STEPWISE.

Some of the more modern selection methods are LASSO, ELASTICNET, and GROUPLASSO. All three of these selection methods apply a penalty to your likelihood to shrink your model parameter estimates down to 0 and find a more parsimonious model representation.

## SELECT= Option

After you specify your SELECTION= option and your selection method, you are then going to use the SELECT= option to specify the criteria. This is the criteria used to determine the order in which effects either enter or leave (or both) at each step of the selection method.

The SELECT= options are shown in Table 6.5.

Table 6.5: SELECT= Options

| SELECT= | Description |
|---|---|
| ADJRSQ | adjusted R-square statistic |
| AIC | Akaike information criterion |
| AICC | corrected Akaike information criterion |
| BIC | Sawa Bayesian information criterion |

| SELECT= | Description |
|---------|-------------|
| CP | Mallow's C(p) statistic |
| CV | predicted residual sum of square with *k*-fold cross validation |
| CVEX | predicted residual sum of square with *k*-fold external cross validation |
| PRESS | predicted residual sum of squares |
| SBC | Schwarz Bayesian information criterion |
| SL | significance level<br><br>The SELECT=SL option must be followed by either of the following options:<br>• SLE= specifies significance level for entry<br>• SLS= specifies significance level for removal |
| VALIDATE | average square error for the validation data. |

> **Tip:** The default value of the SELECT= criterion is SELECT=SBC.
>
> **Tip:** The SELECT= option is not valid with the LAR and LASSO methods.

For example, if we choose SELECT=ADJRSQ, and we are using forward selection, it is going to add parameters into the model iteratively, as long as the adjusted R square continues to increase. The second adjusted R square decreases, the model selection process stops, and the model at the final step will be the model that you deploy.

On the other hand, if you use the AIC option and you are using forward selection, parameters will be iteratively added into the model, as long as the AIC continues to reduce. The second it increases, the model selection process stops.

CHOOSE= Option

You can also use the CHOOSE= option in the MODEL statement to choose the model that yields the best value of the specified criteria from the selection process. The CHOOSE= options are shown in Table 6.6.

Table 6.6: CHOOSE= Options

| SELECT= | Description |
|---------|-------------|
| ADJRSQ | adjusted R-square statistic |
| AIC | Akaike information criterion |
| AICC | corrected Akaike information criterion |
| BIC | Sawa Bayesian information criterion |
| CP | Mallow's C(p) statistic |
| CV | predicted residual sum of square with *k*-fold cross validation |
| CVEX | predicted residual sum of square with *k*-fold external cross validation |

| SELECT= | Description |
|---------|-------------|
| PRESS | predicted residual sum of squares |
| SBC | Schwarz Bayesian information criterion |
| SL | significance level |
| VALIDATE | average square error for the validation data<br><br>This option requires the user to specify a data set in the PROC GLMSELECT statement with the VALDATA= option or use the PARTITION statement to enable the procedure to split the data into training and validation data sets. |

> **Tip:** If no CHOOSE= option is specified, then the model selected is the model at the final step in the selection process.

Behind the scenes when you are doing the selection process, SAS is actually saving model fit statistics. If you use the CHOOSE= AIC option, it actually ignores the model at the final step and simply chooses the model with the best AIC, regardless of where it came in the selection process.

If you ignore the CHOOSE= option, the model selected is the model at the final step. That might not be the same model when you use the CHOOSE= option. Regardless of the final selection process, it will evaluate the specified criteria at each step and choose the best model.

### EFFECTS Statement

Remember when we were creating a Polynomial Regression in PROC REG, we had to first create the quadratic in cubic effects using a DATA step? We can use PROC GLMSELECT to make this process a little bit simpler. Specifically, we can use the EFFECTS statement to bypass creating new variables in the DATA step using the following syntax:

**EFFECT** *name* = *effect-type*(*variables </ options>*) ;

In Program 6.11, we use the EFFECTS statement, and the first thing we do is give it a name. In this case, this will be x_new.

**Program 6.11: EFFECTS Statement in PROC GLMSELECT**
```
proc glmselect data=paper outdesign=des;
    effect x_new = polynomial(amount / degree=5); ❶
    model strength = x_new / selection=none; ❷
run;quit;
```

❶  x_new represents a new set of predictors that the EFFECT statement is creating, and then we will set that equal to an effect type. In this case, we to set it equal to polynomial, but you could also use splines. In parentheses, when we specify the keyword polynomial, give it the variable amount, which is the predictor. After the forward slash we will say degree= to 5. We want to create polynomial regressors for the amount variable up to degree 5, and those will be contained in the x_new variable.

❷  In the MODEL statement, we specify strength and set it equal to the new set of regressors, x_new. Here, we are not doing the selection process, so we will say selection= to none. We just want to fit a polynomial model up to degree 5. If you wanted to alter more than one variable, you can simply pass a list to the polynomial effect type, and be sure to use the outdesign= to option. This is going to create the design matrix or a new SAS data set according to the model that you have created. So in this case it is going to create a new SAS data set with all regressors up to degree 5 without needing to use a DATA step.

If you use the EFFECTS statement in PROC GLMSELECT, it creates a macro variable representing the predictors that you have specified. In this case, in Program 6.11, &_glsmod is representing X, $X^2$, $X^3$, $X^3$, all the way to $X^5$. We can pass that macro variable into a MODEL statement in PROC REG as shown in Program 6.12. If you are passing the variable in to PROC REG, make sure your data set is the OUTPUT data set from the out design option from PROC GLMSELECT. Remember, we called it des, for design matrix.

**Program 6.12: PROC REG Using Macro Variable from Program 6.11**

```
proc reg data=des;
    model y = &_glsmod;
run;quit;
```

In Programs 6.11 and 6.12, we use PROC GLMSELECT to create new regressors and a new SAS data set, and then pass that information to PROC REG to do a Polynomial Regression. We could have stayed in PROC GLMSELECT to do this, but in PROC REG we can get more graphics. If you use the EFFECTS statement to create a set of variables in PROC GLMSELECT and you also do an effects selection process, the new macro variable and SAS data set that it creates will only have the predictors from the final model selection.

So, for example, if it deleted the amount to the fourth and amount to the fifth power in a backward effect selection, the new macro variable and the output data set des would only have the variables amount, amount squared, and amount cubed, which is very convenient.

## Generalized Linear Models

The previous section covered linear models, and now we are going to move on, both in models and procedures. We are going to create generalized linear models now. This is when we are assuming that the response is not Gaussian, but we are going to do the exact same thing. We are going to create models, create statistical graphics, and save other information, create tables, reports, and so on.

In R, we would use the GLM function for the generalized linear model as shown in Figure 6.2. Remember, when you are using the GLM function, you need to specify the appropriate distribution family, with the FAMILY= option. In this section, we will talk about logistic regression for binomial data and Poisson regression, but in SAS, we can use the STORE statement just like we have done before, and use that information in PROC PLM to score new data sets

**Figure 6.2: R Script**

```
#Logistic
mylm = glm(Bonus ~ Basement_Area, family=binomial)
anova(mylm); summary(mylm)
par(mfrow=c(2,2)); plot(mylm)

#Poisson
mylm = glm(Satellites ~ weight, family=poisson)
anova(mylm); summary(mylm)
par(mfrow=c(2,2)); plot(mylm)

#Prediction
predict(mylm, newdata=mynew.dataframe)
```

### PROC LOGISTIC

Most likely, the first model you worked with when you learned generalized linear models was logistic regression. The assumption in logistic regression is that the logit has a linear relationship with the predictor variables. For binary data, and of course, for binomial distributions, we have a probability of success. To model binary variables, we want to model the probability of success, and you will notice in the graph on the left side of Figure 6.3, the probability is not linearly associated with its covariates. It's also bounded between 0 and 1.

**Figure 6.3: Logit Transformation**

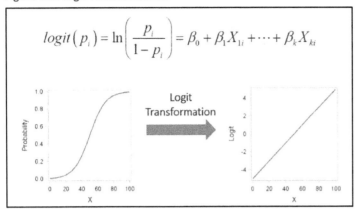

We make the logit transformation and predict the logit, or the log odds. The logit is generally linearly associated with our covariates. Then we can simply specify a linear model as before.

In this section, we will continue to use the ameshousing data set. We use the binary variable for the dependent variable, bonus, and this is simply a value of 1 if the saleprice was greater than $175,000, and a 0 otherwise. We call this variable bonus because home buyers receive a tax incentive for buying a home that is greater than $175,000. To conduct logistic regression, we are going to use the LOGISTIC procedure, so we don't need to specify a family of distributions in this procedure. In the MODEL statement, we specify bonus, and as a best practice in parentheses, you want to tell it what event you are modeling, as shown in the following syntax:

**PROC LOGISTIC DATA=***data-table-name* *<options>*;
   **MODEL** *dependent-variable*(EVENT=) = *effects*;
**RUN**;

In Program 6.13, we want to model the probability of success, or an actual bonus-eligible home, which has a value of 1, and set that equal to just one continuous variable, basement_area.

**Program 6.13: PROC LOGISTIC**

```
proc logistic data=ameshousing;
    model bonus(event='1') = basement_area;
run;
```

**Output 6.13: Results of Program 6.13**

| Model Fit Statistics | | |
|---|---|---|
| Criterion | Intercept Only | Intercept and Covariates |
| AIC | 255.625 | 161.838 |
| SC | 259.329 | 169.246 |
| -2 Log L | 253.625 | 157.838 |

| Testing Global Null Hypothesis: BETA=0 | | | |
|---|---|---|---|
| Test | Chi-Square | DF | Pr > ChiSq |
| Likelihood Ratio | 95.7870 | 1 | < .0001 |
| Score | 65.5624 | 1 | < .0001 |
| Wald | 48.0617 | 1 | < .0001 |

| Odds Ratio Estimates | | | |
|---|---|---|---|
| Effect | Point Estimate | 95% Wald Confidence Limits | |
| Basement_Area | 1.007 | 1.005 | 1.010 |

| Analysis of Maximum Likelihood Estimates | | | | | |
|---|---|---|---|---|---|
| Parameter | DF | Estimate | Standard Error | Wald Chi-Square | Pr > ChiSq |
| Intercept | 1 | -9.7854 | 1.2896 | 57.5758 | < .0001 |
| Basement_Area | 1 | 0.00739 | 0.00107 | 48.0617 | < .0001 |

By default, we get the model fit statistics table and the global null hypothesis tests shown in Output 6.13. One thing to be aware of is that the residual deviance in R is the same as the value 157.838 in SAS. Also, the deviance in R is the likelihood ratio test statistic here at 95.787. There is other information about these tables that you might want to look into as well, but the values will be the same.

Also, by default, we get the odds ratio estimates for each variable in our model. In this case, we only have one, basement_area. This is the odds ratio for a single unit increase in the predictor, which has a point estimate of 1.007. We also get the analysis of maximum likelihood estimates, simply our parameter estimates, standard errors, Wald chi-square test statistic, and our *p*-value.

The odds ratios for a single unit increase in the predictor, basement_area, are not the most meaningful. You are probably not going to want to compare two houses where one is simply one square foot larger in basement area. Use the UNITS statement to specify the units of change for a continuous variable and the CLODDS= option in the MODEL statement to request a confidence interval. As shown in Program 6.14, to change the units of measurement, we will use the UNITS statement and specify the variable, basement_area, equal to 100.

**Program 6.14: PROC LOGISTIC with UNITS Statement and CLODDS= Option**

```
proc logistic data=ameshousing;
    model bonus(event='1') = basement_area
        /clodds=wald;
    units basement_area=100;
run;
```

**Output 6.14: Partial Results of Program 6.14**

| Odds Ratio Estimates and Wald Confidence Intervals | | | | |
|---|---|---|---|---|
| Effect | Unit | Estimate | 95% Confidence Limits | |
| Basement_Area | 100.0 | 2.095 | 1.700 | 2.582 |

| Association of Predicted Probabilities and Observed Responses | | | |
|---|---|---|---|
| Percent Concordant | 89.5 | Somers' D | 0.791 |
| Percent Discordant | 10.4 | Gamma | 0.792 |
| Percent Tied | 0.1 | Tau-a | 0.202 |
| Pairs | 11475 | c | 0.896 |

In the odds ratio estimates in Output 6.14, we get an odds ratio estimate for a home that is 100 square feet larger in basement area. As you can see, the odds for a bonus-eligible house are more than two times the odds with a 100-square-foot difference in basement area. Based on our confidence limits, it is significant. It does not cover a value of 1.

We also get the association of predicted probabilities and observed responses, and this table is just additional output containing model fit. These values are not in the default output in R, so you might not be familiar with them. We will talk more about this first column, the percent concordant, discordant, tied, and pairs in the next section. If you want to look up the statistics for Summers D, Gamma, Tau-a, and C, take a look at the online documentation.

Comparing Pairs

To find the concordant, discordant, and tied pairs, we are going to compare all homes in this data set that are bonus eligible versus not bonus eligible. In this case, that means we are comparing 45 bonus-eligible homes with 255 non-bonus-eligible homes. That is 11,475 total comparisons. But what exactly are we comparing?

In each comparison, we will find the probability of being bonus eligible. In Figure 6.4, we have a bonus-eligible home with 1,200 square feet. We will say the probability of being bonus eligible is 0.28, and the probability of being bonus eligible for the non-bonus-eligible home is 0.02.

**Figure 6.4: Concordant Pair**

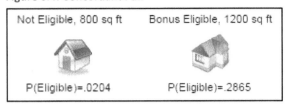

This sorting agrees with our model. We said the probability of being bonus eligible was higher for the actual bonus-eligible home. We will chalk this up to a good model fit and say this is a concordant pair.

On the other hand, if the probability of being bonus eligible for the actual bonus-eligible home is less than the probability of being bonus eligible for the non-bonus-eligible home, this sorting does not agree with our model. We will say the pair shown in Figure 6.5 is a discordant pair.

**Figure 6.5: Discordant Pair**

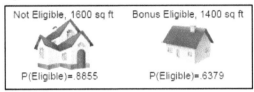

As you can see, we want as many concordant pairs as possible, and as few discordant pairs also. These values are just additional summaries of model fit.

## Effect Selection

Another feature of the LOGISTIC procedure is that you can do effect selection right in the procedure. In the MODEL statement, you can use the SELECTION= option and specify FORWARD, BACKWARD, or STEPWISE model selection. By default, if you are doing FORWARD or BACKWARD selection, the significance level for entry and stay is going to be 0.05, which is different from PROC REG and PROC GLMSELECT.

But again, you can do FORWARD, BACKWARD, and STEPWISE selection right in PROC LOGISTIC. Otherwise, you have to use a different procedure to do more modern effect selection like LASSO, ELASTICNET, and so on.

## PROC GENMOD

Now we are going to move away from PROC LOGISTIC and into the GENMOD procedure. With PROC GENMOD, we can specify any distribution, not just a binomial distribution, but we are going to be doing the exact same things. We are going to run the GENMOD procedure, get graphics, tables, create new data sets, and so on.

In this section, we will look at a new research example. The data come from a study that was conducted about the mating habits of female horseshoe crabs. The population of horseshoe crabs is monitored because they provide a critical food source for migrating birds. Each year, at the end of May and during June, hundreds of thousands of horseshoe crabs emerge from Delaware Bay to lay and fertilize their eggs. Each female horseshoe crab had a male crab resident in her nest. The study investigated factors affecting whether the female horseshoe crab had any other males, called satellites, residing nearby. The response variable for each female horseshoe crab is her number of satellites. The data are stored in Crab.

Figure 6.6 is a partial view of the data. Width and weight are continuous variables. Satellite is a count variable, so as you can tell, we are probably going to be doing Poisson regression. We have two classification variables: color and spine. Color is light medium, medium, dark medium, or dark, but we will use numeric values to indicate those. Spine can be both good, one worn or broken, and both worn or broken.

**Figure 6.6: Female Horseshoe Crab Data**

```
Width    Weight    Color    Spine    Satellites

28.3     3.05       2        3          8
22.5     1.55       3        3          0
26.0     2.30       1        1          9
24.8     2.10       3        3          0
26.0     2.60       3        3          4
23.8     2.10       2        3          0
26.5     2.35       1        1          0
24.7     1.90       3        2          0
23.7     1.95       2        1          0
25.6     2.15       3        3          0
24.3     2.15       3        3          0
25.8     2.65       2        3          0
28.2     3.05       2        3         11
21.0     1.85       4        2          0
26.0     2.30       2        1         14
27.1     2.95       1        1          8
...
```
Color: 1=Light Medium  2=Medium  3=Dark Medium  4=Dark
Spine: 1=Both Good  2=One Worn or Broken  3=Both Worn or Broken

To use PROC GENMOD, we are going to first specify our MODEL statement as shown in the following syntax:

**PROC GENMOD DATA=***data-table-name*;
  **MODEL** *dependent-variable = effects*
    / DIST=*probability-distribution* LINK=*link-function*;
**RUN**;

For the crab data set, we want to predict satellites and will set that equal to the regressor, weight. To specify the distribution, we use the DIST= option the same way we would use the FAMILY= option in R. In Program 6.15, we are sending it to poi for Poisson data. We get all the same default output as PROC LOGISTIC, such as parameter estimates, goodness-of-fit assessments, and so on.

**Program 6.15: PROC GENMOD**
```
proc genmod data=crab;
    model satellites = weight / dist=poi;
run;
```

DIST= Option

There are several different distributions that we can use as options in the MODEL statement as shown in Table 6.7.

**Table 6.7: DIST= Option**

| DIST= | Distribution | Default Link Function |
|---|---|---|
| BINOMIAL | Binomial | Logit |
| GAMMA | Gamma | Inverse |
| GEOMETRIC | Geometric | Log |
| IGAUSSIAN | Inverse Gaussian | Inverse squared |
| MULTINOMIAL | Multinomial | Cumulative logit |
| NEGBIN | Negative Binomial | Log |
| NORMAL | Normal | Identity |
| POISSON | Poisson | Log |
| ZIP | Zero-inflated Poisson | Log/Logit |
| ZINB | Zero-inflated Negative Binomial | Log/Logit |

You can actually specify the binomial distribution to do logistic regression, if you want. Using PROC LOGISTIC is highly recommended instead though, because it knows you are doing a logistic regression and it will give you more relevant graphics. You will notice in Table 6.7 that the right-hand most column is the default link function. When you specify your distribution, it is going to automatically use that appropriate link function. For binomial, it uses the logit. For Poisson, it's going to use the log, and so on.

If, for whatever reason, you wanted to change the link function, just use the LINK= option in the MODEL statement. The LINK= Option options are shown in Table 6.8.

Table 6.8: Link= Option

| LINK= | Link Function |
| --- | --- |
| CUMLL, CCLL | Cumulative Complementary Log-Log |
| CUMLOGIT, CLOGIT | Cumulative Logit |
| CUMPROBIT, CPROBIT | Cumulative Probit |
| CLOGLOG, CLL | Complementary Log-Log |
| IDENTITY, ID | Identity |
| LOG | Log |
| LOGIT | Logit |
| PROBIT | Probit |
| POWER | Power |

**Tip**: The cumulative LINK functions are appropriate only for the multinomial distribution.

For example, if you read an article and you want to change the link function to cumulative logit, you would just specify the appropriate keyword, CUMLOGIT. Most likely, though, you will not be using the link function. You will just be using the default link from the DIST option.

## Mixed Models

In this section we will briefly talk about mixed models and how to create a linear mixed model. We will estimate some variance components and test fixed effects and random effects for significance, but we will be doing all the same things that you have seen in the previous chapters: running a PROC step, generating output, saving new SAS data sets, and so on. We are going to see a lot of the same statements as before.

In R, you probably use the LME4 package, the linear mixed effects model R package, to conduct your mixed models, and then use the LMER function as shown in Figure 6.7. Until now in this book, we have been considering fixed effects only. Fixed effects are those factors whose levels are selected deliberately to evaluate the differences. All levels of interest are in your data set. The researcher is interested in comparing the effects of the factors on the response variable only for those levels included in the study.

**Figure 6.7: R Script**

```
 Source on Save    Q  /  ▾         → Run   ↵   → Source  ▾
#Install the lme4 package
#to compute linear mixed effects models
install.packages("lme4")
library(lme4)

#Create a RCBD model with the LMER function
lmem = lmer(pressure ~ adhesive + (1|toy), data=toys)
summary(lmem)
```

Suppose that you are working for a pharmaceutical company and you are testing three drugs: A, B, and C. These are the only three drugs that you care about. Of course, they did not combine a random process, and these are the only three drugs that you are including in the study. These are fixed effects. A model containing only fixed effects is called a fixed effects model. Models in which some factors are fixed effects and other factors are random effects are called mixed models.

To make this example a mixed model, we need to build in a random effect into our model. Suppose that we want to test our drugs in different clinics. Of course, we can't test our drug in all possible clinics, so the hospital itself is not of direct interest, nor is actually comparing clinic to clinic. We will assume that these clinics are sampled randomly from the population of possible hospitals. To generalize our results beyond the set of clinics included in the study, we will specify these as random.

In some situations, a factor might have a large number of levels and the researcher or data analyst selects a subset of the levels to be included in the study. They represent a sample (although often an imperfect sample) from a population with a probability distribution. The inference about fixed effects from the data analysis applies to all population levels of random effects and not only the subset of levels included in the study. Effects such as these are random effects. For example, in the same drug study, four clinics are randomly selected from a population of clinics in a region. The researcher wants to make an inference for the drug effects across the population of clinics, not only the ones included in the study. Then Clinic is a random effect.

## Mixed Procedure Model

Previously, we have been considering only x beta. Beta are fixed effects, X our fixed effects design matrix. Now, we are including into the model, Z, our random effects design matrix, and gamma are random effects, and we will actually refer to those specific values on the results page as well.

$$Y = X\beta + Z\gamma + \varepsilon$$

We assume that gamma is normally distributed with a mean of 0 and a G-matrix for variance components, and epsilon is normally distributed with a mean of 0 and residual matrix, R. The expected value is the same, just X-Beta, because the expected value of gamma is 0, and if you were to do the matrix multiplication for the variance of y, you would get ZGZ prime plus R. We will call all of this V.

$$E\begin{bmatrix}\gamma \\ \varepsilon\end{bmatrix} = 0 \text{ and } Var\begin{bmatrix}\gamma \\ \varepsilon\end{bmatrix} = \begin{bmatrix}G & 0 \\ 0 & R\end{bmatrix}$$

$$E(y) = X\beta, \quad Var(y) = ZGZ' + R = V$$

There are a few different estimation methods for the covariance parameters in PROC MIXED. We have method of moments and likelihood-based methods, as follows:

- Methods of Moments
  - MIVQUE0
  - Type 1
  - Type 2
  - Type 3

- Likelihood-based Methods
  - ML
  - REML (default)
- For the fixed-effects parameters and standard errors
  - Generalized least squares (GLS) method

MIVQUE performs minimal variance quadratic unbiased estimation of the covariance parameters, so it produces method of moments estimates that are invariant with respect to the fixed effects. That is, the mean squares associated with the random effects are adjusted for the fixed effects. For Type 1, Type 2, and Type 3 method of moments, SAS uses expected mean squares to estimate the variance components.

The likelihood-based methods, in particular ML, can be biased. Most people use REML, residual maximum likelihood, and this is the default method in SAS. It's also the default method in the LME4 package that you probably use in R. REML constructs the likelihood function based on the residuals and obtains maximum likelihood estimates of the variance components from this likelihood. Again, this is the default option because it tends to be the most unbiased.

## PROC MIXED

After you estimate your covariance parameters, you can then estimate your fixed effects parameters and standard errors using the generalized least squares method. PROC MIXED is very similar to the procedures that we have seen thus far, as shown in the following syntax:

**PROC MIXED DATA=***data-table-name*;
   **CLASS** *variables*;
   **MODEL** *dependent-variable= fixed-effects/ solution*;

   **RANDOM** *random-effects/ <options>*;

    **ESTIMATE** *'label' fixed-effect-values| random-effect-values / <options>*;
    **LSMEANS** *fixed-effects/ options*;
**RUN**;

Notice in the syntax that we are building in the RANDOM statement into the model, and as you can expect, we are going to specify all our random effects right in the RANDOM statement. In the MODEL statement, we set the dependent variable equal to only the fixed effects. Your model will look a little bit empty, but again, you only specify your fixed effects in the MODEL statement and your random effects in the RANDOM statement. SAS will then go ahead and combine them to create your complete model.

Let's look at an agricultural example using PROC MIXED. Three seed growth methods are applied to seeds from each of five varieties of turf grass. Six pots are planted with seeds from each method by a variety combination. These 90 pots are randomly placed in a uniform growth chamber and dry matter yields, our response, are measured from clippings at the end of four weeks.

And here is the key sentence: Assume that the five varieties were randomly chosen from a broader population of varieties. Thus, varieties is going to be our random effect and method is going to be our fixed effect. We are only concerned with these specific methods and we want to compare them in our model.

So we are going to do a two-way mixed model. In the equation below, we have mu, the overall mean. Alpha-i is the method effect, b-j is the variety effect, and the inner action, alpha-b, is also going to be random because b is a random effect.

$$y_{ijk} = \mu + \alpha_i + b_j + (\alpha b)_{ij} + \varepsilon_{ijk}$$

We also want to identify our variance components, interaction, variety effect, and error variance components.

$$(\alpha b)_{ij} \sim N(0, \sigma_{\alpha b}^2) \quad b_j \sim N(0, \sigma_b^2) \quad \varepsilon_{ijk} \sim N(0, \sigma^2)$$

First, we use PROC SGPLOT to explore the data in the data set Grass in Program 6.16.

**Program 6.16: PROC SGPLOT**
```
proc sgplot data=sp4r.grass;
    vline variety / group=method stat=mean response=yield;
run;
```

**Output 6.16: Results of Program 6.16**

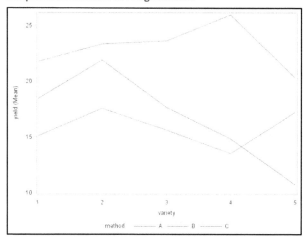

As evidenced in Output 6.16, there seems to be some variability among varieties. In addition, the yield for Method A is largest for all five varieties.

Now we will use PROC MIXED to create a two-way mixed model and use the METHOD=REML option in Program 6.17. (This method reproduces the R package *lmer*.) Remember that the random effects appear only in the RANDOM statement, not the MODEL statement. However, all classification variables, fixed and random effects, are listed in the CLASS statement. Use an LSMEANS statement to compute the least square means for METHOD and use the PDIFF option to evaluate the difference in methods. Finally, use an ESTIMATE statement to compare Method A versus B and C.

**Program 6.17: PROC MIXED**
```
proc mixed data=sp4r.grass method=REML;
    class method variety;
    model yield = method / solution ddfm=kr2;
    random variety method*variety;
    lsmeans method / pdiff;
    estimate 'A vs. B and C' method 1 -.5 -.5;
run;
```

**Output 6.17: Results of Program 6.17**

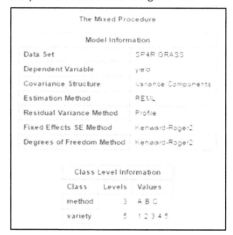

| Dimensions | |
|---|---|
| Covariance Parameters | 3 |
| Columns in X | 4 |
| Columns in Z | 20 |
| Subjects | 1 |
| Max Obs per Subject | 90 |

| Number of Observations | |
|---|---|
| Number of Observations Read | 90 |
| Number of Observations Used | 90 |
| Number of Observations Not Used | 0 |

| Iteration History | | | |
|---|---|---|---|
| Iteration | Evaluations | -2 Res Log Like | Criterion |
| 0 | 1 | 528.89057283 | |
| 1 | 1 | 522.49142693 | 0.00000000 |

Convergence criteria met.

| Covariance Parameter Estimates | |
|---|---|
| Cov Parm | Estimate |
| variety | 0.4285 |
| method*variety | 4.7715 |
| Residual | 19.4347 |

| Fit Statistics | |
|---|---|
| -2 Res Log Likelihood | 522.5 |
| AIC (Smaller is Better) | 528.5 |
| AICC (Smaller is Better) | 528.8 |
| BIC (Smaller is Better) | 527.3 |

| Solution for Fixed Effects | | | | | | |
|---|---|---|---|---|---|---|
| Effect | method | Estimate | Standard Error | DF | t Value | Pr > \|t\| |
| Intercept | | 16.7067 | 1.2863 | 11.9 | 12.99 | <.0001 |
| method | A | 6.3033 | 1.7713 | 8 | 3.56 | 0.0074 |
| method | B | -0.9100 | 1.7713 | 8 | -0.51 | 0.6213 |
| method | C | 0 | | | | |

| Type 3 Tests of Fixed Effects | | | | |
|---|---|---|---|---|
| Effect | Num DF | Den DF | F Value | Pr > F |
| method | 2 | 8 | 9.84 | 0.0070 |

| Estimates | | | | | |
|---|---|---|---|---|---|
| Label | Estimate | Standard Error | DF | t Value | Pr > \|t\| |
| A vs. B and C | 6.7583 | 1.5340 | 8 | 4.41 | 0.0023 |

| Least Squares Means | | | | | | |
|---|---|---|---|---|---|---|
| Effect | method | Estimate | Standard Error | DF | t Value | Pr > \|t\| |
| method | A | 23.0100 | 1.2863 | 11.9 | 17.89 | <.0001 |
| method | B | 15.7967 | 1.2863 | 11.9 | 12.28 | <.0001 |
| method | C | 16.7067 | 1.2863 | 11.9 | 12.99 | <.0001 |

| Differences of Least Squares Means | | | | | | | |
|---|---|---|---|---|---|---|---|
| Effect | method | _method | Estimate | Standard Error | DF | t Value | Pr > \|t\| |
| method | A | B | 7.2133 | 1.7713 | 8 | 4.07 | 0.0036 |
| method | A | C | 6.3033 | 1.7713 | 8 | 3.56 | 0.0074 |
| method | B | C | -0.9100 | 1.7713 | 8 | -0.51 | 0.6213 |

# Other Procedures

At this point, you are probably getting the knack for using SAS procedures. You have seen lots of the same statements and the modeling procedures are very consistent. Once you pick up the syntax, you are going to be able to learn others, especially if you have the modeling background. In this section, we are going to look at a couple of other procedures briefly to get you started in the right direction without going into great detail one each one. Maybe you want to look at generalized linear mixed models, Bayesian models, survival data, multivariate data, or work with time series. What procedures should you start with? Let's find out!

## PROC GLIMMIX

If you want to do generalized linear mixed models, meaning that you want to create a mixed model for a response that is not Gaussian, use the GLIMMIX procedure. Everything is very similar to the other PROCs that we have previously discussed. The only difference is that in the MODEL statement now you are using the DIST= option to specify a probability distribution, and the LINK= option to specify your link, as shown in the following syntax:

**PROC GLIMMIX DATA**=*data-table-name*;
   **CLASS** *variables*;
   **MODEL** *dependent-variable* = *fixed-effects* / SOLUTION
     DIST=*probability-distribution* LINK=*link-function*;
   **RANDOM** *random-effects* / *<options>*;
   **ESTIMATE** '*label*' *fixed-effect-values* | *random-effect-values*
     / *<options>*;
   **LSMEANS** fixed-effects / options;
**RUN**;

In the generalized linear mixed model, you apply a LINK function to the conditional mean $E(y|\gamma)$. The conditional distribution of $y|\gamma$ plays the same role as the distribution of $y$ in the fixed-effects generalized linear model. You apply the same basic strategies for fitting a generalized linear model to $E(y)$ in a fixed effect model to fitting a mixed model to conditional mean $E(y|\gamma)$.

However, to obtain the parameter estimates, you must obtain the marginal log-likelihood function, which is a challenge when you fit generalized linear mixed models (and nonlinear mixed models). By default, the GLIMMIX procedure uses the linearization technique to approximate the generalized linear mixed model as a linear mixed model. Two maximum likelihood methods are also available for fitting generalized linear mixed models in PROC GLIMMIX.

$$p(\theta|x) = \frac{f(x|\theta)\pi(\theta)}{m(x)}$$

The above equation is often expressed as follows:

posterior density=(likelihood*prior)/marginal likelihood

The marginal density of x is an integral defined as follows:

$$\int f(x|\theta)\pi(\theta)d\theta$$

## PROC MCMC

The posterior density or distribution describes the distribution of the parameter of interest with respect to the data and prior. The posterior distribution is necessary for probabilistic prediction and for sequential updating.

Although the name *prior* suggests a temporal relationship, it is feasible for a prior distribution to be decided after seeing the results of the study (for example, empirical Bayes methods. Prior distribution refers to a situation where you assess what the evidence would be if you had no data. This assessment can be made after seeing the data, but there are issues in this.

There is no such thing as the "correct" prior. In fact, researchers suggest using a "community of priors" to describe the range of reasonable opinions.

Even though Bayesian analysis is driven by the prior distribution, it is sometimes not important in the analysis. As the sample size increases, the prior usually is overwhelmed by the likelihood and exerts a negligible influence on the conclusions. However, Bayesian analysis is not based on this assumption.

The development of the posterior distribution might be difficult. The specific problem is carrying out the integrations that are necessary to obtain the posterior distributions of quantities of interest in situations where nonstandard prior distributions are used. For many years, these problems in integration restricted Bayesian applications to rather simple examples involving conjugate priors.

Most Bayesian analyses require sophisticated computations, including the use of simulation methods such as the Monte Carlo methods, to generate samples from the posterior distribution. The basic idea of Monte Carlo is to simulate the sampling process from a defined population repeatedly by using a computer instead of actually drawing multiple samples to estimate the population summaries of the events of interest.

Markov Chain Monte Carlo methods (MCMC) enable researchers to directly sample sequences of values from the posterior distribution of interest, foregoing the need for closed-form analytic solutions. With MCMC, you use these samples to estimate the posterior distribution's quantities of interest. MCMC methods sample successively from a target distribution. Each sample depends on the previous one, hence, the notion of the Markov chain. You can think of a Markov chain applied to sampling as a mechanism that traverses randomly through a target distribution without having any memory of where it was given the immediate past value. Where it moves next is entirely dependent on where it is now.

The Markov chain method is quite successful in modern Bayesian computing. One reason is that if the simulation algorithm is implemented correctly, the Markov chain is guaranteed to converge to the target distribution under rather broad conditions, regardless of the initial values of the parameters. Therefore, the Markov chain is able to improve its approximation to the true distribution at each step in the simulation. Furthermore, the simulation algorithm is easily extensible to models with a large number of parameters or high complexity.

Program 6.18 is an example of a simple linear regression model.

$$Y_i \sim normal(\beta_0 + \beta_1 X_i, \sigma^2)$$

Here we want to estimate three parameters: the intercept, Beta0, the slope, Beta1, and the error, sigma-squared. Use PROC MCMC, specify the number of Monte Carlo simulations, tell SAS what parameters you are working with, give those prior distributions, set a model, and give it a model distribution. SAS will do all the work for you behind the scenes to sample from that posterior.

**Program 6.18: PROC MCMC**
```
proc mcmc data=slrnbi=2000 nmc=10000;
    parms beta0 0 beta1 0;
    parms sigma2 1;
    prior beta0 beta1 ~ normal(mean=0, var=1e6);
    prior sigma2 ~ igamma(shape=2.001, scale=1.001);
    mu=beta0 + beta1*X1;
    model Y ~ normal(mu, var=sigma2);
run;
```

**Output 6.18: Partial Results of Program 6.18**

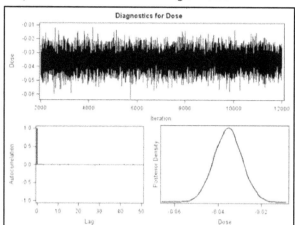

PROC MCMC gives you relevant graphics like the trace plot, the autocorrelation plot, and the density estimates of each parameter.

## PROC LIFETEST

If you are doing survival analyses, you might want to start with PROC LIFETEST. This procedure computes and plots survival function and tests for difference between survival functions. Survival analysis is a collection of specialized methods that are used to analyze data in which time until an event occurs is the response variable of interest. The response variable (often called, in survival analysis, a failure time, survival time, or event time) is usually continuous and can be measured in days, weeks, months, years, and so on. Events can be deaths, onset of disease, marriages, arrests, and so on. What is unique about survival analysis is that even if the subject did not experience an event, the subject's survival time or length of time in the study is taken into account.

Survival analysis is used heavily in clinical and epidemiological follow-up studies. Other fields that use survival analysis methods include sociology, engineering, and economics. Survival analysis is also known as time-to-event analysis, reliability analysis, durability analysis, event history analysis, and lifetime analysis, among others. Regardless of the field, the common objective of a survival analysis study is not only *whether* an event occurred, but also *when* it occurred. For example, subjects who die five years after surgery are different from subjects who die one month after surgery. An analysis that simply counted deaths ignores valuable information about survival time.

Survival analysis can also be used to analyze outcomes other than time. For example, an engineer might want to analyze the amount of mileage until a tire fails or the number of cycles until an engine requires repair. What is common across these studies is that you are analyzing an outcome until an event occurs, and that outcome does not necessarily have to be time.

Survival analysis allows the response variable to be incompletely determined for some subjects. Exact failure time remains unknown. When this occurs, it is called *censoring*. These subjects should not be ignored. The time at which they are observed contributes information to the study. Ignoring them completely adds bias to the estimates of population survival time. They should not be assumed to have the event at the closest observed time point because event times (assuming an event eventually occurs) reported that way would be inaccurately measured.

Censoring is categorized into three main types: *right*, *left*, and *interval*, depending on where the lack of information exists on the timeline relative to the observed follow-up times.

Usually, the first step in the analysis of survival data is to estimate and plot the survival function. The survival function gives the probability that a subject survives longer than some specified time $t$. This can be defined by the formula where $T$ is a random variable for a person's survival time and $t$ is any specific value of interest. At $t=0$, $S(0)=1$ (at the start of the study, because no one experienced the event yet, the probability of surviving past time 0 is 1), while at $t= \infty$, $S(\infty)=0$ (eventually nobody survives, so the survival function theoretically must fall to 0). As *t* increases, S(*t*) never increases and usually decreases. The factors that influence the shape of the survival function are when the subjects experience the event, when the subjects were censored, and the pattern of enrollment in the follow-up study. In practice, the survival function resembles a decreasing step function rather than a smooth curve. Furthermore, because not everyone might experience the event by the end of the study (they are Type I censored), the survival function might not reach 0.

A useful graph in exploratory data analysis is a graph that compares survival functions across groups as shown in Figure 6.8. In the plot at the upper left, the female survival function lies above the male survival function, which means that females had a more favorable survival experience. If the event was death, then at any point in time, the proportion of females estimated to be alive is larger than the proportion of males estimated to be alive.

Figure 6.8: Survival Function Plots

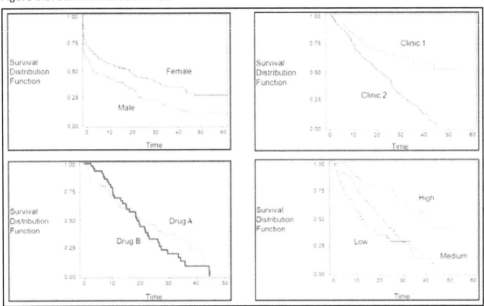

A graph comparing survival functions can also give insight into how time is related to the survival experience across groups. It can indicate interactions with time. In the plot at the upper right, subjects in Clinic 1 have a more favorable survival experience than subjects in Clinic 2. However, the differences between the groups are relatively small in the early time points and become progressively larger in the later time points. Early in the study, both clinics lost a similar proportion of patients. However, as the study progressed, the patients in Clinic 1 had much longer survival times compared to the patients in Clinic 2.

## PROC PHREG

If you are comfortable with survival data, check out the PHREG procedure. The PHREG procedure performs regression analysis of survival data based on the Cox proportional hazard model.

Figure 6.9: PROC PHREG Output

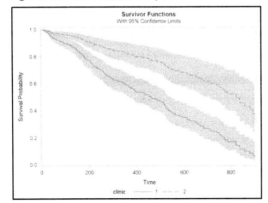

In many situations, either the true form of the hazard function is unknown, or it is so complex that the distributions covered in PROC LIFEREG do not adequately describe your data. This is a problem in parametric models because one of the assumptions is that the true form of the underlying hazard function is correctly specified. Therefore, the parameter estimates of the survival model might be biased if the wrong distribution is specified.

This problem was addressed in 1972 by the British statistician Sir David Cox in a paper called "Regression Models and Life Tables." In his paper, Cox proposed a model (now called the Cox proportional hazards model) that does not require that the distribution of survival times be known. It is a semi-parametric model because it makes a parametric assumption concerning the effect of the predictor variables on the hazard function. (It assumes that the predictor variables act multiplicatively on the hazard function.) However, the model makes no assumption regarding the nature of the hazard function. For example, the model does not assume that the hazard function is constant (the exponential model), or that it follows the form specified in a Weibull model or any other parametric model.

The Cox model is extremely popular because, in many instances, the modeling goal of survival data is to characterize how the distribution of survival times changes as a function of the predictor variables. For example, suppose a clinical trial was designed to test whether one drug therapy improves the survival of AIDS patients when compared to another drug therapy. The primary importance of the survival model is to estimate parameters that compare the survival experience of the two treatment groups. The description of the underlying distribution of survival time is not important. Therefore, the actual form of the baseline hazard function is not important.

Another reason that the Cox model is popular is because the model is as efficient in estimating and testing regression coefficients as the parametric models even when the distribution is correctly specified. When the distribution of survival times is incorrectly specified, the Cox model is more efficient than the parametric models.

The Cox model also uses only the rank ordering of the event and censoring times. This property makes the model less affected by outliers in the event times than in parametric models.

## Multivariate Analysis Procedures

Multivariate analysis refers to a broad category of statistical methods used when more than one variable at a time is analyzed for a subject. Although many physical and virtual systems studied in scientific and business research are, by their very nature, multivariate (that is, there are many responses influenced by many different variables simultaneously), most analyses are univariate (analyzing only one response at a time) in practice. Examples of common multivariate procedures are as follows:

- PROC FACTOR for factor analysis

- PROC CANCORR for canonical correlation

- PROC CANDISC for canonical discrimination

- PROC DISCRIM, in general, to discriminate between different groups

- PROC PLS for partial least squares

- PROC ARIMA for time series so that you can estimate moving average, autoregressive, seasonal components. Once you create the model, you can then go ahead and forecast.

When in doubt, search for a procedure in the documentation at https://support.sas.com/en/documentation.html. Also, check out some of the free videos at support.sas.com/training. These are great resources for learning additional SAS syntax.

# Exercises

1. Which statements are correct? Select all that apply.
   a. The PLM procedure uses the model specified by the STORE statement.
   b. PROC REG uses a CLASS statement to specify categorical variables.
   c. The PLM procedure SCORE statement keywords provide interval output.
   d. The PLM procedure scores new data sets.

2. Choose the correct statements. Select all that apply.
   a. The CLASS statement is equivalent to the as.factor() function in R.
   b. The MEANS statement provides the same default output as PROC MEANS.
   c. The ADJUST= option in the LSMEANS statement is used to adjust for multiple comparisons.
   d. The SOLUTION option in the MODEL statement is used to display parameter estimates.

3. The GLMSELECT procedure can be used to create a regression model, a polynomial regression model, an ANOVA model, an ANCOVA model, and to conduct stepwise model selection.
   a. True
   b. False

4. Consider a logistic regression model where the binary response is whether a person is a dog owner. You sample 140 people and find that 95 people are dog owners. How many total concordant and discordant pairs are considered?
   a. 140
   b. 95*45 = 4275
   c. (95*45)/140 = 30.53
   d. 95*45*140 = 598500

5. Logistic regression can be conducted in both PROC LOGISTIC and PROC GENMOD.
   a. True
   b. False

1. **Fitting a Regression Model**

   Percentage of body fat, age, weight, height, and 10 body circumference measurements were recorded for 252 men by Dr. Roger W. Johnson of Calvin College in Minnesota. The data are in the **BodyFat** data set, which consists of the following variables:

   | | |
   |---|---|
   | **Case** | Case number |
   | **PctBodyFat2** | Percent body fat using Siri's equation (495/density -450) |
   | **Age** | Age in years |
   | **Weight** | Weight in pounds |
   | **Height** | Height in inches |
   | **Neck** | Neck circumference (cm) |
   | **Chest** | Chest circumference (cm) |
   | **Abdomen** | Abdomen circumference (cm) |
   | **Hip** | Hip circumference (cm) |
   | **Thigh** | Thigh circumference (cm) |
   | **Knee** | Knee circumference (cm) |
   | **Ankle** | Ankle circumference (cm) |
   | **Biceps** | Extended biceps circumference (cm) |
   | **Forearm** | Forearm circumference (cm) |
   | **Wrist** | Wrist circumference (cm) |

a.   Generate PROC CORR output for the variables **Height**, **Neck**, **Chest**, and **Weight**. Which variables are highly correlated with **Weight**?

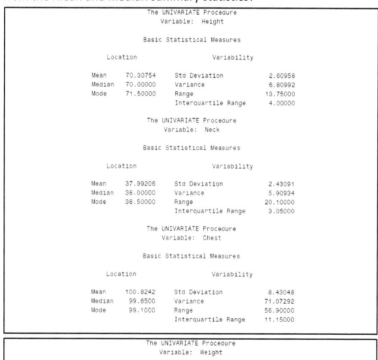

b.   Generate PROC UNIVARIATE output with the same variables. Use the ODS SELECT statement to request only the BasicMeasures table. Do any of the variables appear to be skewed judging only from the mean and median summary statistics?

c. Use PROC SGSCATTER to plot **Weight** by **Height**, **Neck**, and **Chest** separately. Add the regression line to each plot. Does each variable appear to be linearly associated with **Weight**?

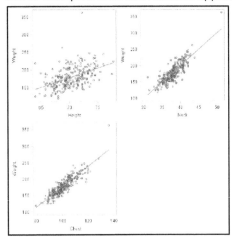

d. Use PROC REG to create a multiple linear regression model with **Weight** as the dependent variable and **Height**, **Neck**, and **Chest** as independent variables. Use the ODS SELECT statement to request only the tables ANOVA, FitStatistics, and ParameterEstimates. Use the OUTPUT statement to create a new data set with the predicted and residual values. Which variables are statistically significant for this model?

```
                          The REG Procedure
                            Model: MODEL1
                      Dependent Variable: Weight

                          Analysis of Variance

                               Sum of          Mean
  Source              DF      Squares        Square    F Value    Pr > F

  Model                3       196216         65405     788.25    <.0001
  Error              248        20578      82.97585
  Corrected Total    251       216794


            Root MSE              9.10911    R-Square     0.9051
            Dependent Mean      178.92440    Adj R-Sq     0.9039
            Coeff Var             5.09104

                          Parameter Estimates

                        Parameter      Standard
  Variable      DF       Estimate         Error    t Value    Pr > |t|

  Intercept      1     -366.66231      16.07211     -22.81      <.0001
  Height         1        2.96912       0.23287      12.75      <.0001
  Neck           1        2.87083       0.39287       7.31      <.0001
  Chest          1        2.25905       0.11015      20.51      <.0001
```

e. Use PROC UNIVARIATE to create a histogram with a normal density estimate and a Q-Q plot compared to a normal distribution of the residuals. Use the ODS SELECT statement to request only the histogram and Q-Q plot. Do the residuals appear to be normally distributed?

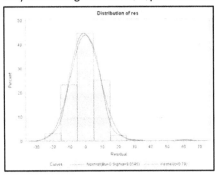 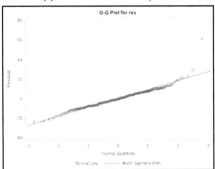

2. **Predicting New Data**
   a. Rerun the model from Exercise 1, but this time use a STORE statement to save the model.
   b. The data set **Newdata_Bodyfat_Reg** contains five new observations. Use PROC PLM to score the new data. Use the PREDICTED keyword in the SCORE statement and save the scored data set as **Pred_Newdata_Bodyfat**.
   c. Print the predicted values from the scored data set and the response and independent variables.

```
Obs    Weight    Height    Neck    Chest    Predicted

 1     179.00    68.00     39.1    103.3    180.847
 2     200.50    69.75     41.3    111.4    210.657
 3     140.25    68.25     33.9     86.0    127.579
 4     148.75    70.00     35.5     86.7    138.950
 5     151.25    67.75     34.5     90.2    137.305
```

3. **Fitting an ANOVA Model**

   The data set **Cars** contains information about a sample of 1993 model cars from the *1993 Cars Annual Auto Issue* published by *Consumer Reports* and from *Pace New Car and Truck 1993 Buying Guide*. The data set consists of the following variables:

   | | |
   |---|---|
   | **Make** | Name of the manufacturer |
   | **Model** | Name of the model |
   | **Type** | Vehicle type (Hybrid, SUV, Sedan, Sports, Truck, or Wagon) |
   | **Origin** | Vehicle origin (Asia, Europe, or USA) |
   | **DriveTrain** | Drivetrain type (All, Front, or Rear) |
   | **Invoice** | Invoice |
   | **MSRP** | Manufacturer's suggested retail price |
   | **EngineSize** | Engine displacement size in liters |
   | **Cylinders** | Number of Cylinders |
   | **Horsepower** | Maximum horsepower |
   | **MPG_City** | Average city miles per gallon (EPA rating) |
   | **MPG_Highway** | Average highway miles per gallon (EPA rating) |
   | **Weight** | Weight of vehicle in pounds |
   | **Wheelbase** | Wheelbase in inches |
   | **Length** | Length of the vehicle in inches |

   a. Generate a frequency table for the variable **Type**. Are the counts of each vehicle in this sample evenly distributed?

```
                           The FREQ Procedure

                                        Cumulative      Cumulative
   Type        Frequency     Percent     Frequency        Percent

   Hybrid          3          0.70           3             0.70
   SUV            60         14.02          63            14.72
   Sedan         262         61.21         325            75.93
   Sports         49         11.45         374            87.38
   Truck          24          5.61         398            92.99
   Wagon          30          7.01         428           100.00
```

   b. Use PROC UNIVARIATE to analyze the **MPG_Highway** variable. Request only the Moments table and the histogram plot with a density estimate. Does **MPG_Highway** appear to be normally distributed?

```
                                Moments

   N                      428        Sum Weights            428
   Mean             26.8434579       Sum Observations      11489
   Std Deviation     5.74120072      Variance          32.9613857
   Skewness          1.25239527      Kurtosis           6.04561068
   Uncorrected SS        322479      Corrected SS       14074.5117
   Coeff Variation   21.3877092      Std Error Mean     0.27751141
```

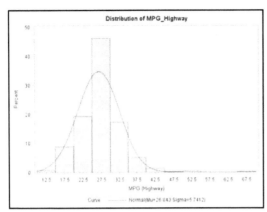

c. Use PROC GLM to create a one-way ANOVA model. Use **MPG_Highway** as the dependent variable and **Type** as the independent variable. Use the PLOTS(ONLY)= option in the PROC GLM statement to request only the ANCOVA plot and use the hybrid vehicle as the reference category. Use the SOLUTION and CLPARM options in the MODEL statement to view parameter estimates and confidence limits. Identify the least squares means (LS-means). Use the ADJUST=TUKEY option and the PDIFF and CL options in the LSMEANS statement. Finally, use the ESTIMATE statement to see whether there is a significant difference in **MPG_Highway** for **SUV** versus **Truck**. Are all parameter estimates statistically significant? Are **SUV** and **Truck** significantly different?

Partial PROC GLM Output

| Source | DF | Sum of Squares | Mean Square | F Value | Pr > F |
|---|---|---|---|---|---|
| Model | 5 | 6743.47900 | 1348.69580 | 77.64 | <.0001 |
| Error | 422 | 7331.03268 | 17.37212 | | |
| Corrected Total | 427 | 14074.51168 | | | |

| Parameter | Estimate | Standard Error | t Value | Pr > |t| | 95% Confidence Limits | |
|---|---|---|---|---|---|---|
| SUV vs Truck | -0.50000000 | 1.00666449 | -0.50 | 0.6197 | -2.47870110 | 1.47870110 |

4. **Fitting an ANCOVA Model**

   a. Extend the ANOVA model above to an ANCOVA model by adding the **HorsePower** variable into the set of independent variables. First, create a macro variable of the mean value of the **HorsePower** variable.

   ```
   215.8855
   ```

   b. Use PROC GLM to fit an ANCOVA model. Use the PLOTS(ONLY)= option to request only the ANCOVA plot from the GLM procedure. Identify the LS-means for the variable Type. Use the AT option to hold the variable **HorsePower** fixed at the mean and use the ADJUST=TUKEY option. Estimate the significance of the same linear combination as before, **SUV** versus **Truck**. Are all parameter estimates statistically significant? Is **SUV** still significantly different from **Truck**?

Partial PROC GLM Output

| Source | DF | Sum of Squares | Mean Square | F Value | Pr > F |
|---|---|---|---|---|---|
| Model | 11 | 10765.94182 | 978.72198 | 123.06 | <.0001 |
| Error | 416 | 3308.56986 | 7.95329 | | |
| Corrected Total | 427 | 14074.51168 | | | |

| Parameter | Estimate | Standard Error | t Value | Pr > |t| | 95% Confidence Limits | |
|---|---|---|---|---|---|---|
| SUV vs Truck | -0.09692078 | 0.69865201 | -0.14 | 0.8897 | -1.47024909 | 1.27640754 |

5. **Fitting a Logistic Regression Model**

The **Safety** data set is created by an insurance company that wants to relate the safety of vehicles to various features. The data set consists of the following variables:

**Unsafe**  1=Yes, 0=No

**Size**  Size of vehicle (1, 2, or 3)

**Weight**  Weight of Vehicle (1, 2, 3, 4, 5, or 6)

**Region**  Asia or North America

**Type**  Vehicle type (Large, Medium, Small, Sport/Utility, or Sports)

a. Use PROC FREQ to create a table of each variable. What percentage of vehicles in the sample are rated as safe?

The FREQ Procedure

| Unsafe | Frequency | Percent | Cumulative Frequency | Cumulative Percent |
|---|---|---|---|---|
| 0 | 66 | 68.75 | 66 | 68.75 |
| 1 | 30 | 31.25 | 96 | 100.00 |

| Size | Frequency | Percent | Cumulative Frequency | Cumulative Percent |
|---|---|---|---|---|
| 1 | 35 | 36.46 | 35 | 36.46 |
| 2 | 29 | 30.21 | 64 | 66.67 |
| 3 | 32 | 33.33 | 96 | 100.00 |

| Weight | Frequency | Percent | Cumulative Frequency | Cumulative Percent |
|---|---|---|---|---|
| 1 | 1 | 1.04 | 1 | 1.04 |
| 2 | 11 | 11.46 | 12 | 12.50 |
| 3 | 53 | 55.21 | 65 | 67.71 |
| 4 | 26 | 27.08 | 91 | 94.79 |
| 5 | 3 | 3.13 | 94 | 97.92 |
| 6 | 2 | 2.08 | 96 | 100.00 |

| Region | Frequency | Percent | Cumulative Frequency | Cumulative Percent |
|---|---|---|---|---|
| Asia | 35 | 36.46 | 35 | 36.46 |
| N America | 61 | 63.54 | 96 | 100.00 |

| Type | Frequency | Percent | Cumulative Frequency | Cumulative Percent |
|---|---|---|---|---|
| Large | 16 | 16.67 | 16 | 16.67 |
| Medium | 29 | 30.21 | 45 | 46.88 |
| Small | 20 | 20.83 | 65 | 67.71 |
| Sport/Utility | 16 | 16.67 | 81 | 84.38 |
| Sports | 15 | 15.63 | 96 | 100.00 |

b. Use PROC LOGISTIC to model the unsafety of a vehicle with independent variables **Weight**, **Region**, and **Size**. Specify **Region** and **Size** as categorical variables with reference categories *Asia* and *3* respectively. Request only the effect plot for the analysis and use the CLODDS=WALD option in the MODEL statement. Use the ESTIMATE statement to estimate the probability of a vehicle from North America with **Weight**=4 and **Size**=1 as unsafe.

Partial PROC Logistic Output

Analysis of Maximum Likelihood Estimates

| Parameter | | DF | Estimate | Standard Error | Wald Chi-Square | Pr > ChiSq |
|---|---|---|---|---|---|---|
| Intercept | | 1 | 0.0500 | 1.8008 | 0.0008 | 0.9778 |
| Weight | | 1 | -0.6678 | 0.4589 | 2.1176 | 0.1456 |
| Region | N America | 1 | -0.3775 | 0.5624 | 0.4506 | 0.5020 |
| Size | 1 | 1 | 2.6783 | 0.8810 | 9.2422 | 0.0024 |
| Size | 2 | 1 | 0.6582 | 0.9231 | 0.5085 | 0.4758 |

c.  Because the significance of the parameter estimates was weak for the model above, conduct backward selection with a significance level to stay in the model of 0.05. Use ODS SELECT to request only the ModelBuildingSummary, ModelAnova, and ParameterEstimates values of the final model. Which variables were removed from the model?

```
                        Summary of Backward Elimination

                 Effect                  Number         Wald
          Step    Removed      DF           In      Chi-Square    Pr > ChiSq

            1     Region        1            2         0.4506        0.5020
            2     Weight        1            1         2.1565        0.1420


                        Type 3 Analysis of Effects

                                            Wald
          Effect         DF          Chi-Square    Pr > ChiSq
```

```
          Size            2           24.2875        <.0001

                Analysis of Maximum Likelihood Estimates

                                        Standard        Wald
          Parameter     DF    Estimate     Error    Chi-Square    Pr > ChiSq

          Intercept      1     -2.7080    0.7303     13.7505        0.0002
          Size       1   1      3.3585    0.8125     17.0880        <.0001
          Size       2   1      1.1393    0.8803      1.6751        0.1956
```

6.  **Fitting a Generalized Linear Model**

A Survey was undertaken to examine which factors are related to ear infections among swimmers. The response variable is the number of self-diagnosed ear infections reported by the participant. The data are stored in the **EarInfection** data set. The data set consists of the following variables:

**Infections**   Number of self-diagnosed ear infections

**Swimmer**    Frequent or Occasional swimmer

**Location**   Typical swimming location (NonBeach or Beach)

**Age**        Age in years

**Gender**     Gender of swimmer (Male or Female)

> The data were obtained with permission from the OZDATA website. This website is a collection of data sets and is maintained in Australia.

a.  Create a frequency table for the variables **Swimmer, Location, Age, Gender**, and **Infections**. What is the range of the number of infections for swimmers in this sample?

```
                          Cumulative    Cumulative
Swimmer  Frequency  Percent  Frequency   Percent

Freq       143     49.83      143        49.83
Occas      144     50.17      287       100.00


                          Cumulative    Cumulative
Location Frequency  Percent  Frequency   Percent

Beach      147     51.22      147        51.22
NonBeach   140     48.78      287       100.00


                          Cumulative    Cumulative
Age    Frequency  Percent  Frequency   Percent

15        28      9.76        28         9.76
16        26      9.06        54        18.82
17        28      9.76        82        28.57
18        32     11.15       114        39.72
19        26      9.06       140        48.78
20        16      5.57       156        54.36
21        15      5.23       171        59.56
22        16      5.57       187        65.15
23        16      5.57       203        70.73
24        16      5.57       219        76.31
25        12      4.18       231        80.49
26        14      4.88       245        85.37
27        14      4.88       259        90.24
28        15      5.23       274        95.47
29        13      4.53       287       100.00


                          Cumulative    Cumulative
Gender  Frequency  Percent  Frequency   Percent

Female     99     34.49       99        34.49
Male      188     65.51      287       100.00


                          Cumulative    Cumulative
Infections Frequency  Percent Frequency   Percent

0         151     52.61      151        52.61
1          40     13.94      191        66.55
2          39     13.59      230        80.14
3          26      9.06      256        89.20
4          13      4.53      269        93.73
5           5      1.74      274        95.47
6           4      1.39      278        96.86
9           3      1.05      281        97.91
10          3      1.05      284        98.95
11          1      0.35      285        99.30
16          1      0.35      286        99.65
17          1      0.35      287       100.00
```

b.  Request only the BasicMeasures table and a histogram with a normal density estimate from PROC UNIVARIATE for the **Infections** variable. Does this variable appear to be normally distributed?

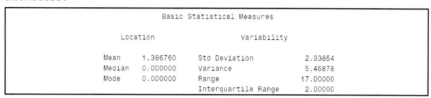

| Basic Statistical Measures | | | |
|---|---|---|---|
| Location | | Variability | |
| Mean | 1.386760 | Std Deviation | 2.33854 |
| Median | 0.000000 | Variance | 5.46878 |
| Mode | 0.000000 | Range | 17.00000 |
| | | Interquartile Range | 2.00000 |

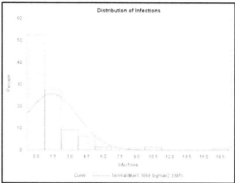

c.  Create a Poisson regression model with **Infections** as the dependent variable and **Swimmer**, **Location**, **Age**, and **Gender** as the independent variables. For the variables **Swimmer**, **Location**, and **Gender** use the reference categories Occas, NonBeach, and Female respectively. Be sure to use the STORE statement to predict the number of Infections using PROC PLM. Which variables are statistically significant?

Partial PROC GENMOD Output

| Analysis Of Maximum Likelihood Parameter Estimates | | | | | | | | |
|---|---|---|---|---|---|---|---|---|
| Parameter | | DF | Estimate | Standard Error | Wald 95% Confidence Limits | | Wald Chi-Square | Pr > ChiSq |
| Intercept | | 1 | 1.3586 | 0.2736 | 0.8224 | 1.8948 | 24.66 | <.0001 |
| Swimmer | Freq | 1 | -0.6086 | 0.1050 | -0.8145 | -0.4028 | 33.59 | <.0001 |
| Location | Beach | 1 | -0.4896 | 0.1048 | -0.6951 | -0.2841 | 21.81 | <.0001 |
| Age | | 1 | -0.0261 | 0.0122 | -0.0500 | -0.0021 | 4.55 | 0.0330 |
| Gender | Male | 1 | -0.0294 | 0.1092 | -0.2433 | 0.1846 | 0.07 | 0.7878 |
| Scale | | 0 | 1.0000 | 0.0000 | 1.0000 | 1.0000 | | |

d.  Create a new data set with the following observations:

| Swimmer | Location | Age | Gender |
|---|---|---|---|
| Freq | NonBeach | 25 | Female |
| Occas | Beach | 15 | Male |

e.  Use PROC PLM to score the new data set and predict the number of **Infections** on the original data scale. Finally, print the predicted values from the PROC PLM output data set.

| Obs | Swimmer | Location | Age | Gender | Predicted |
|---|---|---|---|---|---|
| 1 | Freq | NonBeach | 25 | Female | 1.10338 |
| 2 | Occas | Beach | 15 | Male | 1.56621 |

# Solutions

1. a, c, and d. The PLM procedure scores new data by using the model saved in the STORE statement of the modeling procedures. The REG procedure is generally used to create models with continuous predictors only. Categorical variables would need to be dummy coded by the user for this procedure. The PLM procedure can generate confidence and prediction limits by using options in the SCORE statement.

2. a, c, and d. The CLASS statement is equivalent to the as.factor function in R because it dummy codes your variables for the model. It creates a column in your design matrix for each unique level of each categorical variable that you specify. As a best practice, use the SOLUTION option in the model statement to print your model parameter estimates. The ADJUST= option is used to control the overall type one error for multiple simultaneous comparisons.

3. a. The GLMSELECT procedure can be used to create all the models in PROC REG and PROC GLM, as well as to conduct stepwise effect selection.

4. b. The number of pairs is equal to the number of success times the number of failures (95*45).

5. a. The GENMOD procedure can be used to create any generalized linear model including logistic regression models. However, the LOGISTIC procedure will generate tables and graphics specific to logistic regression models that PROC GENMOD will not.

1. **Fitting a Regression Model**

   Percentage of body fat, age, weight, height, and 10 body circumference measurements were recorded for 252 men by Dr. Roger W. Johnson of Calvin College in Minnesota. The data are in the **BodyFat** data set, which consists of the following variables:

   | | |
   |---|---|
   | **Case** | Case number |
   | **PctBodyFat2** | Percent body fat using Siri's equation (495/density -450) |
   | **Age** | Age in years |
   | **Weight** | Weight in pounds |
   | **Height** | Height in inches |
   | **Neck** | Neck circumference (cm) |
   | **Chest** | Chest circumference (cm) |
   | **Abdomen** | Abdomen circumference (cm) |
   | **Hip** | Hip circumference (cm) |
   | **Thigh** | Thigh circumference (cm) |
   | **Knee** | Knee circumference (cm) |
   | **Ankle** | Ankle circumference (cm) |
   | **Biceps** | Extended biceps circumference (cm) |
   | **Forearm** | Forearm circumference (cm) |
   | **Wrist** | Wrist circumference (cm) |

   a. Generate PROC CORR output for the variables **Height**, **Neck**, **Chest**, and **Weight**. Which variables are highly correlated with **Weight**?

   ```
   proc corr data=sp4r.bodyfat;
       var height neck chest weight;
   run;
   ```

```
                         The CORR Procedure

         4  Variables:    Height   Neck    Chest   Weight

                        Simple Statistics

Variable       N        Mean      Std Dev      Sum     Minimum     Maximum

Height       252     70.30754     2.60958    17718    64.00000    77.75000
Neck         252     37.99206     2.43091     9574    31.10000    51.20000
Chest        252    100.82421     8.43048    25408    79.30000   136.20000
Weight       252    178.92440    29.38916    45089   118.50000   363.15000
```

```
              Pearson Correlation Coefficients, N = 252
                   Prob > |r| under H0: Rho=0

                      Height        Neck        Chest       Weight

      Height         1.00000     0.32114      0.22683      0.48669
                                  <.0001       0.0003       <.0001

      Neck           0.32114     1.00000      0.78484      0.83072
                      <.0001                   <.0001       <.0001

      Chest          0.22683     0.78484      1.00000      0.89419
                      0.0003      <.0001                    <.0001

      Weight         0.48669     0.83072      0.89419      1.00000
                      <.0001      <.0001       <.0001
```

b. Generate PROC UNIVARIATE output with the same variables. Use the ODS SELECT statement to request only the BasicMeasures table. Do any of the variables appear to be skewed judging only from the mean and median summary statistics?

```
ods select basicmeasures;
proc univariate data=sp4r.bodyfat;
var height neck chest weight;
run;
```

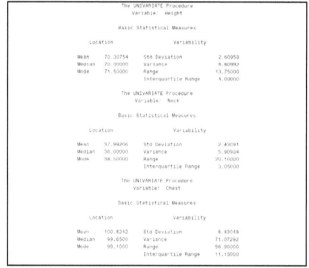

c. Use PROC SGSCATTER to plot **Weight** by **Height**, **Neck**, and **Chest** separately. Add the regression line to each plot. Does each variable appear to be linearly associated with **Weight**?

```
proc sgscatter data=sp4r.bodyfat;
    plot weight * (height neck chest) / reg;
run;
```

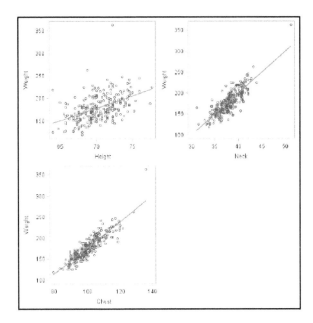

d.  Use PROC REG to create a multiple linear regression model with **Weight** as the dependent variable and **Height**, **Neck**, and **Chest** as independent variables. Use the ODS SELECT statement to request only the tables ANOVA, FitStatistics, and ParameterEstimates. Use the OUTPUT statement to create a new data set with the predicted and residual values. Which variables are statistically significant for this model?

```
ods select anova fitstatistics parameterestimates;
    proc reg data=sp4r.bodyfat;
    model weight = height neck chest;
    output out=sp4r.out predicted=pred residual=res;
run;quit;
```

The REG Procedure
Model: MODEL1
Dependent Variable: Weight

Analysis of Variance

| Source | DF | Sum of Squares | Mean Square | F Value | Pr > F |
|---|---|---|---|---|---|
| Model | 3 | 196216 | 65405 | 788.25 | <.0001 |
| Error | 248 | 20578 | 82.97585 | | |
| Corrected Total | 251 | 216794 | | | |

| | | | | |
|---|---|---|---|---|
| Root MSE | 9.10911 | R-Square | 0.9051 | |
| Dependent Mean | 178.92440 | Adj R-Sq | 0.9039 | |
| Coeff Var | 5.09104 | | | |

Parameter Estimates

| Variable | DF | Parameter Estimate | Standard Error | t Value | Pr > |t| |
|---|---|---|---|---|---|
| Intercept | 1 | -366.66231 | 16.07211 | -22.81 | <.0001 |
| Height | 1 | 2.96912 | 0.23287 | 12.75 | <.0001 |
| Neck | 1 | 2.87083 | 0.39287 | 7.31 | <.0001 |
| Chest | 1 | 2.25905 | 0.11015 | 20.51 | <.0001 |

e.  Use PROC UNIVARIATE to create a histogram with a normal density estimate and a Q-Q plot compared to a normal distribution of the residuals. Use the ODS SELECT statement to request only the histogram and Q-Q plot. Do the residuals appear to be normally distributed?

```
ods select histogram qqplot;
proc univariate data=sp4r.out;
    var res;
    histogram res / normal kernel;
    qqplot res / normal(mu=est sigma=est);
run;
```

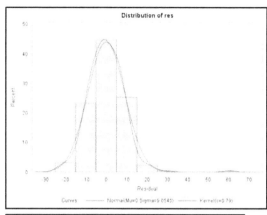

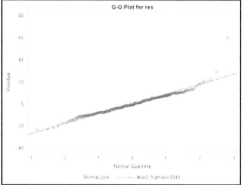

2. **Predicting New Data**

   a. Rerun the model from Exercise 1, but this time use a STORE statement to save the model.

   ```
   proc reg data=sp4r.bodyfat;
       model weight = height neck chest;
       store mymod;
   run;quit;
   ```

   b. The data set **Newdata_Bodyfat_Reg** contains five new observations. Use PROC PLM to score the new data. Use the PREDICTED keyword in the SCORE statement and save the scored data set as **Pred_Newdata_Bodyfat**.

   ```
   proc plm restore=mymod;
       score data=sp4r.newdata_bodyfat_reg
       out=sp4r.pred_newdata_bodyfat predicted;
   run;
   ```

   c. Print the predicted values from the scored data set and the response and independent variables.

   ```
   proc print data=sp4r.pred_newdata_bodyfat;
       var weight height neck chest predicted;
   run;
   ```

   | Obs | Weight | Height | Neck | Chest | Predicted |
   |-----|--------|--------|------|-------|-----------|
   | 1 | 179.00 | 68.00 | 39.1 | 103.3 | 180.847 |
   | 2 | 200.50 | 69.75 | 41.3 | 111.4 | 210.657 |
   | 3 | 140.25 | 68.25 | 33.9 | 86.0 | 127.579 |
   | 4 | 148.75 | 70.00 | 35.5 | 86.7 | 138.950 |
   | 5 | 151.25 | 67.75 | 34.5 | 90.2 | 137.305 |

3. **Fitting an ANOVA Model**

The data set **Cars** contains information about a sample of 1993 model cars from the *1993 Cars Annual Auto Issue* published by *Consumer Reports* and from *Pace New Car and Truck 1993 Buying Guide*. The data set consists of the following variables:

| | |
|---|---|
| **Make** | Name of the manufacturer |
| **Model** | Name of the model |
| **Type** | Vehicle type (Hybrid, SUV, Sedan, Sports, Truck, or Wagon) |
| **Origin** | Vehicle origin (Asia, Europe, or USA) |
| **DriveTrain** | Drivetrain type (All, Front, or Rear) |
| **Invoice** | Invoice |
| **MSRP** | Manufacturer's suggested retail price |
| **EngineSize** | Engine displacement size in liters |
| **Cylinders** | Number of Cylinders |
| **Horsepower** | Maximum horsepower |
| **MPG_City** | Average city miles per gallon (EPA rating) |
| **MPG_Highway** | Average highway miles per gallon (EPA rating) |
| **Weight** | Weight of vehicle in pounds |
| **Wheelbase** | Wheelbase in inches |
| **Length** | Length of the vehicle in inches |

a. Generate a frequency table for the variable **Type**. Are the counts of each vehicle in this sample evenly distributed?

```
proc freq data=sp4r.cars;
    table type;
run;
```

```
                     The FREQ Procedure

                                 Cumulative   Cumulative
Type     Frequency    Percent    Frequency     Percent

Hybrid          3       0.70             3        0.70
SUV            60      14.02            63       14.72
Sedan         262      61.21           325       75.93
Sports         49      11.45           374       87.38
Truck          24       5.61           398       92.99
Wagon          30       7.01           428      100.00
```

b. Use PROC UNIVARIATE to analyze the **MPG_Highway** variable. Request only the Moments table and the histogram plot with a density estimate. Does **MPG_Highway** appear to be normally distributed?

```
ods select moments histogram;
    proc univariate data=sp4r.cars;
    var mpg_highway;
    histogram mpg_highway / normal;
run;
```

```
                     The UNIVARIATE Procedure
            Variable:  MPG_Highway  (MPG (Highway))

                            Moments

N                         428    Sum Weights                 428
Mean               26.8434579    Sum Observations          11489
Std Deviation      5.74120072    Variance             32.9613857
Skewness           1.25239527    Kurtosis             6.04561068
Uncorrected SS         322479    Corrected SS         14074.5117
Coeff Variation    21.3877092    Std Error Mean       0.27751141
```

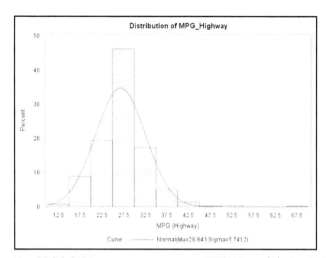

c.  Use PROC GLM to create a one-way ANOVA model. Use **MPG_Highway** as the dependent variable and **Type** as the independent variable. Use the PLOTS(ONLY)= option in the PROC GLM statement to request only the ANCOVA plot and use the hybrid vehicle as the reference category. Use the SOLUTION and CLPARM options in the MODEL statement to view parameter estimates and confidence limits. Identify the least squares means (LS-means). Use the ADJUST=TUKEY option and the PDIFF and CL options in the LSMEANS statement. Finally, use the ESTIMATE statement to see whether there is a significant difference in **MPG_Highway** for **SUV** versus **Truck**. Are all parameter estimates statistically significant? Are **SUV** and **Truck** significantly different?

```
proc glm data=sp4r.cars plots(only)=boxplot;
    class type (ref='Hybrid');
    model mpg_highway = type / solution clparm;
    lsmeans type / adjust=tukey pdiff cl;
    estimate 'SUV vs Truck' type 1 0 0 -1 0 0;
run;quit;
```

```
                          The GLM Procedure

                        Class Level Information

           Class        Levels   Values

           Type              6    SUV Sedan Sports Truck Wagon Hybrid

              Number of Observations Read         428
              Number of Observations Used         428
```

```
                    Dependent Variable: MPG_Highway    MPG (Highway)

                                          Sum of
         Source                  DF       Squares     Mean Square   F Value   Pr > F

         Model                    5     6743.47900     1348.69580     77.64   <.0001

         Error                  422     7331.03268       17.37212

         Corrected Total        427    14074.51168


                    R-Square    Coeff Var    Root MSE    MPG_Highway Mean

                    0.479127    15.52701     4.167987         26.84346


         Source                  DF     Type I SS     Mean Square   F Value   Pr > F

         Type                     5    6743.478998    1348.695800    77.64    <.0001


         Source                  DF    Type III SS    Mean Square   F Value   Pr > F

         Type                     5    6743.478998    1348.695800    77.64    <.0001


                                          Standard
Parameter             Estimate             Error     t Value   Pr > |t|     95% Confidence Limits

Intercept          56.00000000 B        2.40638840    23.27    <.0001     51.26999968  60.73000032
Type    SUV        -35.50000000 B       2.46581434   -14.40    <.0001    -40.34680804 -30.65319196
Type    Sedan      -27.37022901 B       2.42012622   -11.31    <.0001    -32.12723240 -22.61322562
Type    Sports     -30.51020408 B       2.47895907   -12.31    <.0001    -35.38284942 -25.63755875
Type    Truck      -35.00000000 B       2.55236033   -13.71    <.0001    -40.01692295 -29.98307705
Type    Wagon      -28.10000000 B       2.52384144   -11.13    <.0001    -33.06086618 -23.13913382
Type    Hybrid       0.00000000 B           .            .        .             .            .

NOTE: The X'X matrix has been found to be singular, and a generalized inverse was used to solve
      the normal equations.  Terms whose estimates are followed by the letter 'B' are not
      uniquely estimable.
```

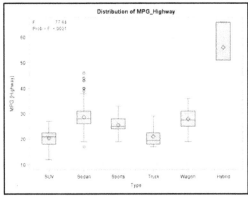

Distribution of MPG_Highway

```
                         Least Squares Means
              Adjustment for Multiple Comparisons: Tukey-Kramer

                          MPG_Highway      LSMEAN
               Type          LSMEAN        Number

               SUV        20.5000000          1
               Sedan      28.6297710          2
               Sports     25.4897959          3
               Truck      21.0000000          4
               Wagon      27.9000000          5
               Hybrid     56.0000000          6


               Least Squares Means for effect Type
               Pr > |t| for H0: LSMean(i)=LSMean(j)

               Dependent Variable: MPG_Highway

 i/j       1          2          3          4          5          6

  1                 <.0001     <.0001     0.9963     <.0001     <.0001
  2      <.0001                <.0001     <.0001     0.9443     <.0001
  3      <.0001     <.0001                0.0003     0.1280     <.0001
  4      0.9963     <.0001     0.0003                <.0001     <.0001
  5      <.0001     0.9443     0.1280     <.0001                <.0001
  6      <.0001     <.0001     <.0001     <.0001     <.0001
                          MPG_Highway
               Type         LSMEAN      95% Confidence Limits
```

```
SUV        20.500000      19.442340    21.557660
Sedan      28.629771      28.123630    29.135912
Sports     25.489796      24.319424    26.660167
Truck      21.000000      19.327692    22.672308
Wagon      27.900000      26.404243    29.395757
Hybrid     56.000000      51.270000    60.730000

         Least Squares Means for Effect Type

              Difference        Simultaneous 95%
              Between        Confidence Limits for
       i    j    Means        LSMean(i)-LSMean(j)

       1    2    -8.129771     -9.837539    -6.422003
       1    3    -4.989796     -7.287355    -2.692237
       1    4    -0.500000     -3.381944     2.381944
       1    5    -7.400000    -10.068162    -4.731838
       1    6   -35.500000    -42.559293   -28.440707

Adjustment for Multiple Comparisons: Tukey-Kramer

         Least Squares Means for Effect Type

              Difference        Simultaneous 95%
              Between        Confidence Limits for
       i    j    Means        LSMean(i)-LSMean(j)

       2    3     3.139975      1.282775     4.997175
       2    4     7.629771      5.084970    10.174572
       2    5     0.729771     -1.570120     3.029662
       2    6   -27.370229    -34.298723   -20.441735
       3    4     4.489796      1.516864     7.462728
       3    5    -2.410204     -5.176394     0.355986
       3    6   -30.510204    -37.607128   -23.413280
       4    5    -6.900000    -10.167817    -3.632183
       4    6   -35.000000    -42.307062   -27.692938
       5    6   -28.100000    -35.325416   -20.874584

Dependent Variable: MPG_Highway    MPG (Highway)

                        Standard
Parameter      Estimate    Error   t Value  Pr > |t|   95% Confidence Limits

SUV vs Truck  -0.50000000  1.00566449  -0.50   0.6197  -2.47870110   1.47870110
```

4. **Fitting an ANCOVA Model**

   a. Extend the ANOVA model above to an ANCOVA model by adding the **HorsePower** variable into the set of independent variables. First, create a macro variable of the mean value of the **HorsePower** variable.

   ```
   proc sql;
       select mean(horsepower) into :hp_mean from sp4r.cars;
   quit;
   ```

   ```
   215.8855
   ```

   b. Use PROC GLM to fit an ANCOVA model. Use the PLOTS(ONLY)= option to request only the ANCOVA plot from the GLM procedure. Identify the LS-means for the variable Type. Use the AT option to hold the variable **HorsePower** fixed at the mean and use the ADJUST=TUKEY option. Estimate the significance of the same linear combination as before, **SUV** versus **Truck**. Are all parameter estimates statistically significant? Is **SUV** still significantly different from **Truck**?

   ```
   proc glm data=sp4r.cars plots(only)=ancovaplot;
       class type (ref='Hybrid');
       model mpg_highway = type|horsepower / solution clparm;
       lsmeans type / at horsepower=&hp_mean
               adjust=tukey pdiff cl;
       estimate 'SUV vs Truck' type 1 0 0 -1 0 0 type*horsepower
       &hp_mean 0 0 -&hp_mean 0 0;
   run;quit;
   ```

   ```
                    The GLM Procedure

                 Class Level Information

        Class     Levels   Values

        Type        6      SUV Sedan Sports Truck Wagon Hybrid

           Number of Observations Read      428
           Number of Observations Used      428
   ```

Dependent Variable: MPG_Highway    MPG (Highway)

| Source | DF | Sum of Squares | Mean Square | F Value | Pr > F |
|---|---|---|---|---|---|
| Model | 11 | 10765.94182 | 978.72198 | 123.06 | <.0001 |
| Error | 416 | 3308.56986 | 7.95329 | | |
| Corrected Total | 427 | 14074.51168 | | | |

| R-Square | Coeff Var | Root MSE | MPG_Highway Mean |
|---|---|---|---|
| 0.764925 | 10.50594 | 2.820158 | 26.84346 |

| Source | DF | Type I SS | Mean Square | F Value | Pr > F |
|---|---|---|---|---|---|
| Type | 5 | 6743.478998 | 1348.695800 | 169.58 | <.0001 |
| Horsepower | 1 | 3699.837286 | 3699.837286 | 465.20 | <.0001 |
| Horsepower*Type | 5 | 322.625534 | 64.525107 | 8.11 | <.0001 |

| Source | DF | Type III SS | Mean Square | F Value | Pr > F |
|---|---|---|---|---|---|
| Type | 5 | 653.3927903 | 130.6785581 | 16.43 | <.0001 |
| Horsepower | 1 | 272.6094049 | 272.6094049 | 34.28 | <.0001 |
| Horsepower*Type | 5 | 322.6255340 | 64.5251068 | 8.11 | <.0001 |

| Parameter | | Estimate | Standard Error | t Value | Pr > |t| |
|---|---|---|---|---|---|
| Intercept | | 94.22157434 B | 10.03894199 | 9.39 | <.0001 |
| Type | SUV | -64.05940099 B | 10.16284659 | -6.30 | <.0001 |
| Type | Sedan | -55.15403535 B | 10.05608869 | -5.48 | <.0001 |
| Type | Sports | -61.56306301 B | 10.12406223 | -6.08 | <.0001 |
| Type | Truck | -62.82986720 B | 10.28016825 | -6.11 | <.0001 |

| Parameter | | 95% Confidence Limits | |
|---|---|---|---|
| Intercept | | 74.48819768 | 113.95495100 |
| Type | SUV | -84.03633480 | -44.08246718 |
| Type | Sedan | -74.92111698 | -35.38695372 |
| Type | Sports | -81.46375905 | -41.66236696 |
| Type | Truck | -83.03741819 | -42.62231620 |

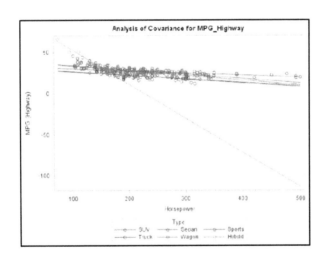

| Parameter | | Estimate | Standard Error | t Value | Pr > |t| |
|---|---|---|---|---|---|
| Type | Wagon | -55.28132488 B | 10.17751744 | -5.43 | <.0001 |
| Type | Hybrid | 0.00000000 B | . | . | . |
| Horsepower | | -0.41545190 B | 0.10767414 | -3.86 | 0.0001 |
| Horsepower*Type | SUV | 0.37447865 B | 0.10787191 | 3.47 | 0.0006 |
| Horsepower*Type | Sedan | 0.36369176 B | 0.10771002 | 3.38 | 0.0008 |
| Horsepower*Type | Sports | 0.39022444 B | 0.10776347 | 3.62 | 0.0003 |
| Horsepower*Type | Truck | 0.36923229 B | 0.10809315 | 3.42 | 0.0007 |
| Horsepower*Type | Wagon | 0.35854339 B | 0.10798664 | 3.32 | 0.0010 |
| Horsepower*Type | Hybrid | 0.00000000 B | . | . | . |

| Parameter | | 95% Confidence Limits | |
|---|---|---|---|
| Type | Wagon | -75.28709693 | -35.27555284 |
| Type | Hybrid | . | |
| Horsepower | | -0.62710512 | -0.20379867 |

| | | |
|---|---|---|
| Horsepower*Type SUV | 0.16243668 | 0.58652063 |
| Horsepower*Type Sedan | 0.15196801 | 0.57541550 |
| Horsepower*Type Sports | 0.17839563 | 0.60205326 |
| Horsepower*Type Truck | 0.15675543 | 0.58170915 |
| Horsepower*Type Wagon | 0.14627590 | 0.57081088 |
| Horsepower*Type Hybrid | . | . |

The GLM Procedure
Least Squares Means at Horsepower=215.5855
Adjustment for Multiple Comparisons: Tukey-Kramer

| Type | MPG_Highway LSMEAN | LSMEAN Number |
|---|---|---|
| SUV | 21.3166445 | 1 |
| Sedan | 27.8932754 | 2 |
| Sports | 27.2122700 | 3 |
| Truck | 21.4135653 | 4 |
| Wagon | 26.6545290 | 5 |
| Hybrid | 4.5315343 | 6 |

Least Squares Means for effect Type
Pr > |t| for H0: LSMean(i)=LSMean(j)

Dependent Variable: MPG_Highway

| i/j | 1 | 2 | 3 | 4 | 5 | 6 |
|---|---|---|---|---|---|---|
| 1 | | <.0001 | <.0001 | 1.0000 | <.0001 | 0.8125 |
| 2 | <.0001 | | 0.7970 | <.0001 | 0.2596 | 0.5072 |
| 3 | <.0001 | 0.7970 | | <.0001 | 0.9750 | 0.5414 |
| 4 | 1.0000 | <.0001 | <.0001 | | <.0001 | 0.8091 |
| 5 | <.0001 | 0.2596 | 0.9750 | <.0001 | | 0.5692 |
| 6 | 0.8125 | 0.5072 | 0.5414 | 0.8091 | 0.5692 | |

| Type | MPG_Highway LSMEAN | 95% Confidence Limits | |
|---|---|---|---|
| SUV | 21.315645 | 20.555637 | 22.075652 |
| Sedan | 27.893275 | 27.542081 | 28.244470 |
| Sports | 27.212270 | 26.225452 | 28.199088 |
| Truck | 21.413565 | 20.269704 | 22.557427 |
| Wagon | 26.654529 | 25.582575 | 27.726483 |
| Hybrid | 4.531534 | -21.883643 | 30.946912 |

Least Squares Means for Effect Type

| i | j | Difference Between Means | Simultaneous 95% Confidence Limits for LSMean(i)-LSMean(j) | |
|---|---|---|---|---|
| 1 | 2 | -6.576631 | -7.796069 | -5.357193 |
| 1 | 3 | -5.895626 | -7.709609 | -4.081442 |
| 1 | 4 | -0.095921 | -2.097200 | 1.903356 |
| 1 | 5 | -5.337884 | -7.251807 | -3.423962 |
| 1 | 6 | 16.785110 | -21.705315 | 55.275535 |

Least Squares Means at Horsepower=215.5855
Adjustment for Multiple Comparisons: Tukey-Kramer

Least Squares Means for Effect Type

| i | j | Difference Between Means | Simultaneous 95% Confidence Limits for LSMean(i)-LSMean(j) | |
|---|---|---|---|---|
| 2 | 3 | 0.681005 | -0.844623 | 2.206633 |
| 2 | 4 | 6.479710 | 4.736897 | 8.222523 |
| 2 | 5 | 1.238746 | -0.404232 | 2.881725 |
| 2 | 6 | 23.361741 | -15.116163 | 61.839645 |
| 3 | 4 | 5.798705 | 3.598335 | 7.999075 |
| 3 | 5 | 0.557741 | -1.564430 | 2.679912 |
| 3 | 6 | 22.680736 | -15.820606 | 61.182078 |
| 4 | 5 | -5.240964 | -7.524265 | -2.957662 |
| 4 | 6 | 16.882031 | -21.628529 | 55.392591 |
| 5 | 6 | 22.122995 | -16.383176 | 60.629166 |

The GLM Procedure

Dependent Variable: MPG_Highway   MPG (Highway)

| Parameter | Estimate | Standard Error | t Value | Pr > |t| | 95% Confidence Limits | |
|---|---|---|---|---|---|---|
| SUV vs Truck | -0.09692076 | 0.69865201 | -0.14 | 0.8897 | -1.47024909 | 1.27640754 |

5. **Fitting a Logistic Regression Model**

The **Safety** data set is created by an insurance company that wants to relate the safety of vehicles to various features. The data set consists of the following variables:

**Unsafe**  1=Yes, 0=No

**Size**  Size of vehicle (1, 2, or 3)

**Weight**  Weight of Vehicle (1, 2, 3, 4, 5, or 6)

**Region**  Asia or North America

**Type**  Vehicle type (Large, Medium, Small, Sport/Utility, or Sports)

a. Use PROC FREQ to create a table of each variable. What percentage of vehicles in the sample are rated as safe?

```
proc freq data=sp4r.safety;
run;
```

```
                        The FREQ Procedure

                                   Cumulative    Cumulative
     Unsafe   Frequency   Percent   Frequency     Percent

        0         66       68.75        66         68.75
        1         30       31.25        96        100.00

                                   Cumulative    Cumulative
     Size     Frequency   Percent   Frequency     Percent

        1         35       36.46        35         36.46
        2         29       30.21        64         66.67
        3         32       33.33        96        100.00

                                   Cumulative    Cumulative
     Weight   Frequency   Percent   Frequency     Percent

        1          1        1.04         1          1.04
        2         11       11.46        12         12.50
        3         53       55.21        65         67.71
        4         26       27.08        91         94.79
        5          3        3.13        94         97.92
        6          2        2.08        96        100.00

                                   Cumulative    Cumulative
     Region     Frequency  Percent   Frequency     Percent

     Asia          35       36.46        35         36.46
     N America     61       63.54        96        100.00

                                   Cumulative    Cumulative
     Type       Frequency  Percent   Frequency     Percent

     Large          16      16.67        16         16.67
     Medium         29      30.21        45         46.88
     Small          20      20.83        65         67.71
     Sport/Utility  16      16.67        81         84.38
     Sports         15      15.63        96        100.00
```

b. Use PROC LOGISTIC to model the unsafety of a vehicle with independent variables **Weight**, **Region**, and **Size**. Specify **Region** and **Size** as categorical variables with reference categories *Asia* and *3* respectively. Request only the effect plot for the analysis and use the CLODDS=WALD option in the MODEL statement. Use the ESTIMATE statement to estimate the probability of a vehicle from North America with **Weight**=4 and **Size**=1 as unsafe.

```
proc logistic data=sp4r.safety plots(only)=effect;
    class region(ref='Asia') size(ref='3') / param=ref;
    model unsafe(event='1') = weight region size /
        clodds=wald;
    estimate 'My Estimate' intercept 1 weight 4 region 1
        size 1 0 / e alpha=.05 ilink;
run;
```

```
                   The LOGISTIC Procedure

                      Model Information

     Data Set                      WORK.SAFETY
     Response Variable             Unsafe
     Number of Response Levels     2
     Model                         binary logit
     Optimization Technique        Fisher's scoring

          Number of Observations Read        96
          Number of Observations Used        96

                      Response Profile

          Ordered                   Total
           Value     Unsafe       Frequency

             1          0             66
             2          1             30
```

```
                    Probability modeled is Unsafe=1.

                      Class Level Information

                                        Design
              Class      Value        Variables

              Region     Asia             0
                         N America        1

              Size       1                1      0
                         2                0      1
                         3                0      0

                    Model Convergence Status

          Convergence criterion (GCONV=1E-8) satisfied.
```

```
                       Model Fit Statistics

                                       Intercept
                            Intercept      and
              Criterion       Only      Covariates

              AIC            121.249       94.004
              SC             123.813      106.826
              -2 Log L       119.249       84.004

             Testing Global Null Hypothesis: BETA=0

      Test              Chi-Square     DF     Pr > ChiSq

      Likelihood Ratio     35.2441      4       <.0001
      Score                32.8219      4       <.0001
      Wald                 23.9864      4       <.0001

                   Type 3 Analysis of Effects

                                 Wald
              Effect     DF    Chi-Square    Pr > ChiSq

              Weight      1      2.1176        0.1456
              Region      1      0.4506        0.5020
              Size        2     15.3370        0.0005
```

```
              Analysis of Maximum Likelihood Estimates

                                   Standard      Wald
      Parameter          DF  Estimate   Error  Chi-Square  Pr > ChiSq

      Intercept           1    0.0500   1.8008    0.0008     0.9778
      Weight              1   -0.6678   0.4589    2.1176     0.1456
      Region  N America   1   -0.3775   0.5624    0.4506     0.5020
      Size    1           1    2.6783   0.8810    9.2422     0.0024
      Size    2           1    0.6582   0.9231    0.5085     0.4758


         Association of Predicted Probabilities and Observed Responses

              Percent Concordant    81.9   Somers' D   0.696
              Percent Discordant    12.3   Gamma       0.739
              Percent Tied           5.8   Tau-a       0.302
              Pairs                 1980   c           0.848
```

```
                 Odds Ratio Estimates and Wald Confidence Intervals

        Effect                       Unit     Estimate     95% Confidence Limits

        Weight                      1.0000      0.513      0.209      1.261
        Region N America vs Asia    1.0000      0.686      0.228      2.064
        Size   1 vs 3               1.0000     14.560      2.590     81.857
        Size   2 vs 3               1.0000      1.931      0.316     11.793

                           Estimate Coefficients

                   Parameter              Region      Size      Row1

                   Intercept: Unsafe=0                           1
                   Weight                                        4
                   Region N America     N America                1
                   Size 1                            1           1
                   Size 2                            2

                                   Estimate

                                                                         Error of
Label         Estimate    Error  z Value  Pr > |z|  Alpha   Lower   Upper   Mean    Mean

My Estimate   -0.3204    0.6916   -0.46    0.6432    0.05  -1.6759  1.0352  0.4206  0.1685

                                   Estimate

                                          Lower      Upper
                          Label           Mean       Mean

                          My Estimate    0.1576     0.7379
```

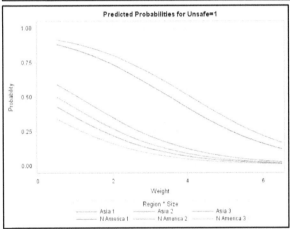

*Predicted Probabilities for Unsafe=1*

c.  Because the significance of the parameter estimates was weak for the model above, conduct
    backward selection with a significance level to stay in the model of 0.05. Use ODS SELECT to
    request only the ModelBuildingSummary, ModelAnova, and ParameterEstimates values of the
    final model. Which variables were removed from the model?

```
ods select modelbuildingsummary modelanova
      parameterestimates;
proc logistic data=sp4r.safety;
    class region(ref='Asia') size(ref='3') / param=ref;
    model unsafe(event='1') = weight region size /
        selection=backward sls=.05 clodds=wald;
run;
```

```
                         The LOGISTIC Procedure

                     Summary of Backward Elimination

                  Effect             Number        Wald
          Step    Removed    DF        In      Chi-Square   Pr > ChiSq

           1      Region     1         2          0.4506     0.5020
           2      Weight     1         1          2.1565     0.1420

                     Type 3 Analysis of Effects

                                       Wald
                  Effect    DF     Chi-Square   Pr > ChiSq
```

```
              Size        2      24.2875       <.0001

                Analysis of Maximum Likelihood Estimates

                                  Standard        Wald
       Parameter     DF    Estimate    Error   Chi-Square   Pr > ChiSq

       Intercept      1    -2.7080    0.7303    13.7505      0.0002
       Size      1    1     3.3585    0.8125    17.0880      <.0001
       Size      2    1     1.1393    0.8803     1.6751      0.1956
```

6. **Fitting a Generalized Linear Model**

   A Survey was undertaken to examine which factors are related to ear infections among swimmers. The response variable is the number of self-diagnosed ear infections reported by the participant. The data are stored in the **EarInfection** data set. The data set consists of the following variables:

   | | |
   |---|---|
   | **Infections** | Number of self-diagnosed ear infections |
   | **Swimmer** | Frequent or Occasional swimmer |
   | **Location** | Typical swimming location (NonBeach or Beach) |
   | **Age** | Age in years |
   | **Gender** | Gender of swimmer (Male or Female) |

   > The data were obtained with permission from the OZDATA website. This website is a collection of data sets and is maintained in Australia.

   a. Create a frequency table for the variables **Swimmer, Location, Age, Gender**, and **Infections**. What is the range of the number of infections for swimmers in this sample?

   ```
   proc freq data=sp4r.earinfection;
        tables swimmer location age gender infections;
   run;
   ```

   ```
                              The FREQ Procedure

                                           Cumulative   Cumulative
            Swimmer    Frequency   Percent   Frequency    Percent

            Freq          143      49.83       143        49.83
            Occas         144      50.17       287       100.00


                                           Cumulative   Cumulative
            Location   Frequency   Percent   Frequency    Percent

            Beach         147      51.22       147        51.22
            NonBeach      140      48.78       287       100.00

                                           Cumulative   Cumulative
            Age     Frequency   Percent   Frequency    Percent

             15        28        9.76        28          9.76
             16        26        9.06        54         18.82
             17        28        9.76        82         28.57
             18        32       11.15       114         39.72
   ```

| | | | Cumulative | Cumulative |
|---|---|---|---|---|
| 19 | 26 | 9.06 | 140 | 48.78 |
| 20 | 16 | 5.57 | 156 | 54.36 |
| 21 | 15 | 5.23 | 171 | 59.58 |
| 22 | 16 | 5.57 | 187 | 65.16 |
| 23 | 16 | 5.57 | 203 | 70.73 |
| 24 | 16 | 5.57 | 219 | 76.31 |
| 25 | 12 | 4.18 | 231 | 80.49 |
| 26 | 14 | 4.88 | 245 | 85.37 |
| 27 | 14 | 4.88 | 259 | 90.24 |
| 28 | 15 | 5.23 | 274 | 95.47 |
| 29 | 13 | 4.53 | 287 | 100.00 |

| Gender | Frequency | Percent | Cumulative Frequency | Cumulative Percent |
|---|---|---|---|---|
| Female | 99 | 34.49 | 99 | 34.49 |
| Male | 188 | 65.51 | 287 | 100.00 |

| Infections | Frequency | Percent | Cumulative Frequency | Cumulative Percent |
|---|---|---|---|---|
| 0 | 151 | 52.61 | 151 | 52.61 |
| 1 | 40 | 13.94 | 191 | 66.55 |
| 2 | 39 | 13.59 | 230 | 80.14 |
| 3 | 26 | 9.06 | 256 | 89.20 |
| 4 | 13 | 4.53 | 269 | 93.73 |
| 5 | 5 | 1.74 | 274 | 95.47 |
| 6 | 4 | 1.39 | 278 | 96.86 |
| 9 | 3 | 1.05 | 281 | 97.91 |
| 10 | 3 | 1.05 | 284 | 98.95 |
| 11 | 1 | 0.35 | 285 | 99.30 |
| 16 | 1 | 0.35 | 286 | 99.65 |
| 17 | 1 | 0.35 | 287 | 100.00 |

b.  Request only the BasicMeasures table and a histogram with a normal density estimate from PROC UNIVARIATE for the **Infections** variable. Does this variable appear to be normally distributed?

```
ods select basicmeasures histogram;
proc univariate data=sp4r.earinfection;
    var infections;
    histogram infections / normal;
run;
```

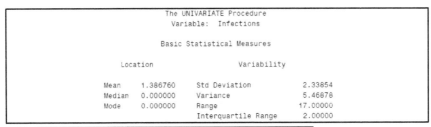

The UNIVARIATE Procedure
Variable: Infections

Basic Statistical Measures

| Location | | Variability | |
|---|---|---|---|
| Mean | 1.386760 | Std Deviation | 2.33854 |
| Median | 0.000000 | Variance | 5.46878 |
| Mode | 0.000000 | Range | 17.00000 |
| | | Interquartile Range | 2.00000 |

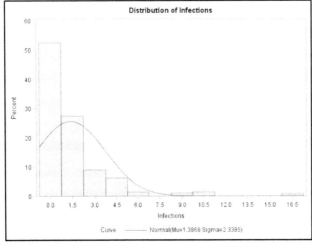

c. Create a Poisson regression model with **Infections** as the dependent variable and **Swimmer**, **Location**, **Age**, and **Gender** as the independent variables. For the variables **Swimmer**, **Location**, and **Gender** use the reference categories Occas, NonBeach, and Female respectively. Be sure to use the STORE statement to predict the number of Infections using PROC PLM. Which variables are statistically significant?

```
proc genmod data=sp4r.earinfection;
    class swimmer(ref='Occas') location(ref='NonBeach')
        gender(ref='Female') / param=ref;
    model infections = swimmer location age gender /
        dist=poisson type3;
    store mymod;
run;
```

The GENMOD Procedure

Model Information

| | |
|---|---|
| Data Set | WORK.EARINFECTION |
| Distribution | Poisson |
| Link Function | Log |
| Dependent Variable | Infections |

| | |
|---|---|
| Number of Observations Read | 287 |
| Number of Observations Used | 287 |

Class Level Information

| Class | Value | Design Variables |
|---|---|---|
| Swimmer | Freq | 1 |
| | Occas | 0 |
| Location | Beach | 1 |
| | NonBeach | 0 |
| Gender | Female | 0 |
| | Male | 1 |

Criteria For Assessing Goodness Of Fit

| Criterion | DF | Value | Value/DF |
|---|---|---|---|
| Deviance | 282 | 760.0060 | 2.6951 |
| Scaled Deviance | 282 | 760.0060 | 2.6951 |
| Pearson Chi-Square | 282 | 963.5838 | 3.4170 |
| Scaled Pearson X2 | 282 | 963.5838 | 3.4170 |
| Log Likelihood | | -235.6148 | |
| Full Log Likelihood | | -566.2004 | |
| AIC (smaller is better) | | 1142.4008 | |
| AICC (smaller is better) | | 1142.6143 | |
| BIC (smaller is better) | | 1160.6982 | |

Algorithm converged.

Analysis Of Maximum Likelihood Parameter Estimates

| Parameter | | DF | Estimate | Standard Error | Wald 95% Confidence Limits | | Wald Chi-Square | Pr > ChiSq |
|---|---|---|---|---|---|---|---|---|
| Intercept | | 1 | 1.3586 | 0.2736 | 0.8224 | 1.8948 | 24.66 | <.0001 |
| Swimmer | Freq | 1 | -0.6086 | 0.1050 | -0.8145 | -0.4028 | 33.59 | <.0001 |
| Location | Beach | 1 | -0.4896 | 0.1048 | -0.6951 | -0.2841 | 21.81 | <.0001 |
| Age | | 1 | -0.0261 | 0.0122 | -0.0500 | -0.0021 | 4.55 | 0.0330 |
| Gender | Male | 1 | -0.0294 | 0.1092 | -0.2433 | 0.1846 | 0.07 | 0.7878 |
| Scale | | 0 | 1.0000 | 0.0000 | 1.0000 | 1.0000 | | |

NOTE: The scale parameter was held fixed.

LR Statistics For Type 3 Analysis

| Source | DF | Chi-Square | Pr > ChiSq |
|---|---|---|---|
| Swimmer | 1 | 35.16 | <.0001 |
| Location | 1 | 22.35 | <.0001 |
| Age | 1 | 4.64 | 0.0312 |
| Gender | 1 | 0.07 | 0.7881 |

d.  Create a new data set with the following observations:

| Swimmer | Location | Age | Gender |
|---------|----------|-----|--------|
| Freq | NonBeach | 25 | Female |
| Occas | Beach | 15 | Male |

```
data sp4r.newdata_inf;
    input Swimmer $ Location $ Age Gender $;
    datalines;
Freq NonBeach 25 Female
Occas Beach 15 Male
;run;
```

e.  Use PROC PLM to score the new data set and predict the number of **Infections** on the original data scale. Finally, print the predicted values from the PROC PLM output data set.

```
proc plm restore=mymod;
    score data=sp4r.newdata_inf out=sp4r.scores / ilink;
run;
```

```
                        The PLM Procedure

                        Store Information

        Item Store              WORK.EARPRED
        Data Set Created From   WORK.EARINFECTION
        Created By              PROC Genmod
        Date Created            13OCT15:09:52:16
        Response Variable       Infections
        Link Function           Log
        Distribution            Poisson
        Class Variables         Swimmer Location Gender
        Model Effects           Intercept Swimmer Location Age Gender
```

```
proc print data=sp4r.scores;
run;
```

```
    Obs   Swimmer   Location   Age   Gender   Predicted

     1     Freq     NonBeach    25   Female    1.10338
     2     Occas    Beach       15   Male      1.56621
```

# Chapter 7: Interactive Matrix Language (IML)

## Introduction

This chapter is all about SAS Interactive Matrix Language (SAS IML). Because R is a matrix language, it is important to know how to accomplish similar matrix-based tasks in SAS. The IML procedure enables you to completely customize analyses and run code interactively.

We will start with the basics of working in the IML procedure, such as creating and printing matrices. Then, we will practice using built-in SAS modules and creating our own. Next, we will explore more of the nuances of working with SAS IML from an R user's perspective. In particular, you will learn how to read in SAS data sets to an IML matrix to run customized analyses and how to save those results in a SAS data set. Finally, we will learn how to run Monte Carlo simulations.

## The Basics of IML

In this section, we will review the basics of working in the interactive matrix language. We want to use matrix algebra to customize our statistical analyses, so in the equation below, for example, we have a hypothesized model.

$$Y = \beta_0 + \beta_1 X_1 + ... + \beta_k X_k + \varepsilon$$

We could pass the model to PROC REG or PROC GLM. But instead, in this chapter, we will do all the matrix algebra to find our parameter estimates. In the equation below, the beta hat vector is x transpose x inverse, x transpose y, where x is the design matrix and y is the vector of observed values.

$$\hat{\beta} = (X^T X)^- X^T Y$$

## PROC IML

In this section, we will create a matrix manually. We will do some elementwise operations, matrix operations. We will access and pull out elements of matrices, and finally, we will talk about some reduction operators, so how to use basic functions like MAX, SUM, and COLMEANS.

Here is the general form of the PROC IML step:

**PROC IML;**
   *IML syntax*
**QUIT;**

> To save space, the examples in this chapter tend to omit the PROC IML; and QUIT; lines.

We start with the PROC IML statement, and then we have all of our IML syntax. This could be many, many, many lines of code. Once we are done working in the interactive matrix language, we run a single QUIT statement to get out, but everything between PROC IML and QUIT is going to be a matrix. Very different from what we have seen in the previous chapters.

PROC IML can be used interactively or in batch mode. Using IML in batch mode entails submitting the PROC IML call, a set of IML statements, and finally a QUIT statement. PROC IML does not require a RUN statement. To use IML in interactive mode, submit the PROC IML call. IML statements can then be submitted one at a time or in groups. When IML is no longer needed, submit the QUIT statement to exit IML.

Brackets, braces, and parentheses have distinct uses in SAS/IML.

- Brackets { } are used for making a matrix from literal values.

- Braces [ ] are used to pull elements out of a matrix.

- Parentheses ( ) are used to specify the order of operations, or as part of a built-in or user-defined function.

To create a matrix by hand, we will simply specify a matrix as shown in Program 7.1. Call it x and set it equal to the following using the brackets. Specify the first row of the matrix (1, 2, 3), followed by a comma to go to the second row of the matrix (4, 5, 6). Now, x is a 2-by-3 matrix.

**Program 7.1: Matrix with Numerical Data**

```
PROC IML;
x = {1 2 3,
     4 5 6}

QUIT;
```

We can also enter in character data as well. In Program 7.2, we have a vector that is 3-by-1, which is all character data: Jordan, Baker, and finally Man. The only thing to remember about character data is the size is the number of characters for the longest word, in this case six characters.

**Program 7.2: Matrix with Character Data**

```
PROC IML;
x = {"Jordan",
     "Baker",
     "Man}
QUIT;
```

SAS/IML matrices must contain either character or numeric elements. A matrix cannot contain both types of elements. Numeric elements are stored in double-precision floating point-format using eight bytes. Elements of character matrices can be from 1 to 32,767 bytes long. Matrices are referenced by valid SAS names. Names can be from 1 to 32 characters long, beginning with a letter or an underscore and continuing with any combination of letters, underscores, or digits.

If you assigned character values to a matrix, and then you assign an element, the value 2 not enclosed in quotation marks, the element contains the character '2', not the floating point numeric representation of 2, because matrices cannot be of mixed type.

The length of each element in a character matrix is determined dynamically to be the length of the longest element. For example, if you assign the value dog to element 1 of a matrix and the value horse to element 2, then the first element is five bytes long, and the last two bytes are blank characters. If you later change element 2 to cat, the length of elements remains five unless a longer element was assigned. The LENGTH statement can be used to determine the length of each element in a character matrix.

If you want to view a matrix, use the PRINT statement because, remember, SAS does not have a command-line interpreter. In Program 7.3, we have the x equal to the 2-by-3 matrix from Program 7.1. If we want to print it to the results page, we just say PRINT X. There are lots of other options that you can use in the PRINT statement.

**Program 7.3: PRINT Statement**

```
PROC IML;
x = {1 2 3,
     4 5 6}
print x;
QUIT;
```

If you don't want to use an assignment statement, meaning you don't want to set your matrix equal to a variable (in this case, x), and you just want to print something, use parentheses in your PRINT statement as shown in Program 7.4.

**Program 7.4: Alternative PRINT Statement**

```
print ( {1 2 3,
         4 5 6});
```

Everything between the parentheses in your PRINT statement will be printed to the results page. It doesn't have to just be a matrix. You can also do mathematical operations, for example, but again, you have to use parentheses if you are not assigning it to a variable.

## Accessing Matrix Elements

Figure 7.1 shows how to create and access matrices in R. SAS has a few similarities to R in the way it accesses elements.

**Figure 7.1: R Script**

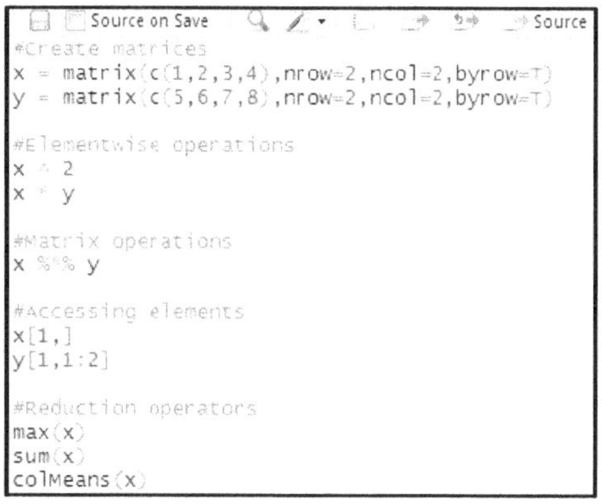

In SAS, we also have our X matrix, which we created and is 2 by 3.

$$X = \begin{bmatrix} 1 & 2 & 3 \\ 4 & 5 & 6 \end{bmatrix}$$

To access matrix elements, we use the following syntax:

*matrix-name[row,column]*;

For example, X[2,1] goes to matrix X and pulls out the second row, first column element, which is 4.

If we leave the COLUMN or ROW argument open, it simply takes out all the columns or rows, as shown in the following syntax:

*matrix[row,]*;
*matrix[,column]*;

For example, X[2, ] goes into the second row and pulls out the entire row (4, 5, 6).

Finally, to find dimensions, use NROW and NCOL on the matrix, as shown in the following syntax:

*nrow(matrix)*;
*ncol(matrix)*;

In practice, we need to use an assignment statement such as D1=nrow(X) or D1=ncol(X). Otherwise, we would have to use a PRINT statement followed by the parentheses.

> **Tip:** SAS/IML does not have a dim() function.

## Creating a Sequence

The index operator in SAS is identical to R, as shown in the following syntax:

*value1:value2*;

X = 1:5; creates a sequence from 1 to 5 using the colon, and it simply creates the row vector.

You can also use the DO function with following syntax:

*vector* = **DO**(*start,stop,increment*);

X = do(2, 10, 2); goes from 2 to 10, by an increment of 2 to create a row vector [2 4 6 8 10].

## Basic Operators

Table 7.1 shows a comparison of basic operators that are used in both SAS and R.

**Table 7.1: Basic Operators**

| Description | SAS Operator | R Operator |
|---|---|---|
| Elementwise | +, -, #, /, ## | +, -, *, /, ^ |
| Matrix Multiplication | * | %*% |
| Matrix Exponentiation | ** | |
| Transpose | t() or ` | t() |
| Horizontal Concatenation | \|\| | rbind() |

| Description | SAS Operator | R Operator |
|---|---|---|
| Vertical Concatenation | // | cbind() |

The first thing you should notice in Table 7.1 is the star operator in red. In R, the star does elementwise multiplication, but SAS uses the hashtag. R uses the double hashtag to exponentiate a matrix, but SAS uses the single star operator to do matrix multiplication. You need to be very conscious of which software language you are working in because if you are in R and you use the star, it's elementwise operations. If you use the star in SAS, it's matrix multiplication.

## Comparison Operators

Comparison operators perform elementwise comparisons and produce a new matrix that contains only 0s and 1s. If an element comparison is true, the corresponding element of the new matrix is 1. If the comparison is not true, the corresponding element is 0. Unlike in Base SAS, in IML, you cannot use the mnemonic equivalents (GT, LT, GE, LE, NE, EQ). Table 7.2 shows comparison operators in both SAS and R.

**Table 7.2: Comparison Operators**

| Description | SAS Operator | R Operator |
|---|---|---|
| Less than | < | < |
| Less than or equal to | <= | <= |
| Equal to | = | == |
| Not equal to | ^= | != |
| Greater than | > | > |
| Greater than or equal to | >= | >= |

As you can see in Table 7.2, the comparison operators in SAS are similar to R, specifically the less than, less or equal to, greater than, or greater than or equal to. Again, just like we saw in Chapter 2, we do not use the double equal sign, and we do not use the exclamation point for not equal to. Here, we just have the up caret for not equal to.

Using these comparison operators is very similar to R. See the following example:

```
Z = {2 7, 3 5} > {4 6, 5 8}
```

$$\begin{bmatrix} 2 & 7 \\ 3 & 5 \end{bmatrix} > \begin{bmatrix} 4 & 6 \\ 5 & 8 \end{bmatrix} = \begin{bmatrix} 0 & 1 \\ 0 & 0 \end{bmatrix}$$

Here, we are specifying a matrix Z, and saying, "Is this matrix greater than the following matrix?" Each element of the matrix is compared and returns a binary result. Because two is not greater than four, it returns a zero. Seven is greater than six, so it returns a one, and so on.

## Implicit Looping

Some matrix operations can be performed on matrices that are not conformable to the operation. We have actually been doing matrix and scalar operations in R all along. For example, see the following operation:

$$\begin{bmatrix} 2 & 6 \\ 5 & 9 \end{bmatrix} + 3 = \begin{bmatrix} 5 & 9 \\ 8 & 12 \end{bmatrix}$$

In this case, if we add a scalar to a matrix, it is simply going to add 3 to every element of the matrix.

The next two operations are new if you have never worked in SAS. The first is matrix and row vector, an example of which is shown in the following operation:

$$\begin{bmatrix} 2 & 6 \\ 5 & 9 \end{bmatrix} - \begin{bmatrix} 5 & 2 \end{bmatrix} = \begin{bmatrix} -3 & 4 \\ 0 & 7 \end{bmatrix}$$

Here we have a 2 by 2 matrix and a 1 by 2 row vector. Notice that we have the same number of columns in each. We can do a matrix in row vector operation, meaning we are going to apply the operation to each row of the matrix. So 2 minus 5 is minus 3, 6 minus 2 is 4, and then we apply the same row vector operation to the next row in the matrix.

If **X** is an *m*-by-*n* matrix, and **Y** is a 1-by-*n* row vector, then the expression **X+Y** evaluates to the addition of **Y** to each row of **X**. This change was introduced to reduce the need for explicit loops and increase the efficiency of this type of calculation.

The second type of operation is matrix and column vector. It works similarly to matrix and row vector, as you can see in the following example:

$$\begin{bmatrix} 2 & 6 \\ 5 & 9 \end{bmatrix} / \begin{bmatrix} 2 \\ 4 \end{bmatrix} = \begin{bmatrix} 1 & 3 \\ 1.25 & 2.25 \end{bmatrix}$$

Notice in this case that we have the same number of rows, so we are going to apply this operation to each column in the matrix. 2 divided by 2 is 1, 5 divided by 4 is 1.25, and then moving on to the second column in the matrix.

## Subscript Reduction Operators

Subscript reduction operators are a good way to find some summary statistics quickly on a matrix. The operators are listed in Table 7.3.

Table 7.3: Subscript Reduction Operators

| Operator | Description |
|---|---|
| + | Sum |
| # | Product |
| <> | Maximum |
| >< | Minimum |
| <:> | Index of maximum |
| >:< | Index of minimum |
| : | Mean |
| ## | Sum of squares |

Let's use the following 3 by 3 matrix as an example:

$$X = \begin{bmatrix} 1 & 2 & 3 \\ 6 & 5 & 9 \\ 7 & 8 & 4 \end{bmatrix}$$

To help you decide whether to specify an operator in the row or column dimension, remember that if a dimension's subscript is missing, that dimension remains unchanged in the new matrix. In the example below, the subscript for the column dimension is missing, so the resulting matrix has the same number of columns, three.

You can use reduction operators to reduce either rows or columns or both. When both rows and columns are reduced, row reduction is done first.

Let's look at a few examples of operations on the example matrix:

- Y=X[+, ]    produces    Y=[14 15 16]
- Y=X[, <>]   produces    Y=[3, 9, 8]
- Y=X[#,]     produces    Y=[42 80 108]
- Y=X[:,]     produces    Y=[14/3 5 16/3]

In the first example operation, the first argument for the rows is the plus symbol followed by a comma, which means we are leaving the column argument open. This is saying we want to sum each row for all columns. So 1 plus 6 plus 7 is 14, 2 plus 5 plus 8 is 15, and so on.

The next example uses the maximum operator, so we want to take the maximum of the columns for each row. The max for the first row is 3, the second row is 9, and so on.

## Modules and Subroutines

In this section, we will learn how to apply a SAS module, or user-defined module, to a matrix and bring back a result. We will also see how to simulate random numbers from probability distributions. We can create random matrices or vectors, just like in R, as shown in Figure 7.2. Then we will use some base R functions like SOLVE, which solves a linear system of equations, or SVD, to do the singular value decomposition. Finally, at the end of the section, you will learn how to create a user-defined function.

**Figure 7.2: R Script**

```
      Source on Save       Q  /  ·              Source
#Random numbers
x = matrix(rnorm(100),nrow=10,ncol=10,byrow=T)
y = rnorm(1000,mean=10,sd=10)

#Base R functions
vec = solve(A,b)
svd(C)

#User-defined functions
add = function(a,b){
  c = a + b
  return(c)
}
```

### Modules

In SAS, the term module is more of an umbrella term that refers to either a function or subroutine, but they both perform a specific task, just like a function in R. IML functions and subroutines perform common operations that would otherwise require many lines of IML code. There are a few differences, though, between a function and a subroutine.

- General form of an IML function:
  *result = function-name(argument-1, argument-2, ...)*;

- General form of an IML subroutine:
  **CALL** *subroutine-name<(argument-1, argument-2, ...)>*;

## Function

First, notice that a function uses an assignment statement. IML functions are not valid without an assignment statement. We need to specify a new variable name (in this case, the result), and set it equal to the function that we are using, and then supply the arguments to actually use the function. Whereas with the subroutine, we do not use the assignment statement. We just run it with a CALL statement.

More importantly, there is a subtle distinction. Functions *return* matrices. Subroutines *create* matrices. We will see the difference going forward.

Again, function modules return only a single matrix. They must have at least one argument and require an assignment statement. Here is an example of a function module:

```
X = {3 4 5,
     2 4 9};
numberRows = nrow(X);
numberCols = ncols(X);
```

We have the X matrix, which is 2 by 3, and we are using the NROW and NCOLS functions. In order for this to be valid, to actually use the built-in function, we are setting it equal to new matrices that we are calling numberRows and numberCols.

## Subroutine

Subroutine modules, on the other hand, do not return a matrix. They create or alter a matrix. They can have no arguments, and they cannot be called in an assignment statement, so you cannot set it equal to a new variable. In the example below, we use the SORT subroutine and call it with the CALL statement.

```
call sort(X);
```

Here we supply the single argument X. It's going to re-sort the matrix X, so the new matrix will be 2 3 4, 4 5 9.

Some subroutines create matrices without an assignment statement. Let's look at an example of using the EIGEN subroutine to create a matrix with the following syntax:

**CALL EIGEN** (*eigenvalues, eigenvectors, matrix*);

Notice that the syntax has three arguments: the eigenvalues, eigenvectors, and matrix. In Program 7.5, we have a 2-by-2 matrix x, and we will run the Eigen subroutine with the CALL statement. Notice that we are only passing it one argument x. The other two arguments, evals and evecs, are the matrices being created.

**Program 7.5: EIGEN Subroutine**

```
x = {1 2,3 4};
call eigen(evals,evecs,x);
print evals evecs;
```

**Output 7.5: Results of Program 7.5**

| evals | | evecs | |
|---|---|---|---|
| 5.3722813 | 0 | -0.415974 | -0.824565 |
| -0.372281 | 0 | -0.909377 | 0.5657675 |

When we do the eigenvalue decomposition, it creates the evals matrix and evecs matrix, which are the eigenvalues and eigenvectors. Then when we run that subroutine, we have access to use them in SAS. Output 7.5 shows the results of printing those new matrices, evals and evecs.

## Random Number Generation Functions

In Chapter 4, we talked about simulating random numbers in a DATA step. Notice in Table 7.4 that the PDF, CDF, and QUANTILE functions are exactly the same. (This table is the same as Table 4.2 in Chapter 4.)

**Table 7.4: PDF, CDF, and QUANTILE Functions with R Counterparts**

| R | SAS |
| --- | --- |
| dnorm(q,mean, sd) | PDF('Normal',q,mean,sd) |
| pnorm(q,mean,sd) | CDF('Normal',q,mean,sd) |
| qnorm(p,mean,sd) | QUANTILE('Normal',p,mean,sd) |

We specify a distribution, either the quantile or the cumulative density, followed by the parameters. The point here is that some of the functions we have already used in DATA steps, you can use directly in IML as well, but be sure to check the documentation.

### J Function

Let's take a closer look at a function. The J function creates a matrix with n rows and p columns, and it fills every element of the new matrix with the same value using the following syntax:

**J**(*nrows,ncols,<value>*)

In Program 7.6, we are creating matrix X with the J function. Of course, it's not case sensitive, so we could use a little j. In parentheses, specify the number of rows 2, the number of columns 3, and fill every element with the value 0. If we leave off the optional value, it will simply fill the matrix with a default value of 1.

**Program 7.6: J Function**
```
X = J(2,3,0)
```

On the surface, the J function might not seem like it is extremely helpful, but in combination with the RANDGEN subroutine, it is very useful.

### RANDGEN Subroutine

The RANDGEN subroutine can be used to fill a matrix with random numbers using the following syntax:

**CALL RANDGEN**(*result, dist-name<,parm1><,parm2><,parm3>*);

The result matrix must be created by the user before calling RANDGEN. RANDGEN produces the number of samples required to fill each cell in the matrix. The result matrix must be numeric and should have a number of cells equal to the desired number of samples. The number of parameters that are specified is dependent on the distribution. For example, specifying the Cauchy distribution does not require any parameters whereas specifying a normal mixture distribution requires three parameters.

To create a matrix with simulated random values, first initialize a matrix with the J function as shown in Program 7.7.

**Program 7.7: RANDGEN Subroutine**
```
X = J(2,3,0);
call randgen(X,"Normal",10,2);
```

You can see that Program 7.7 creates a new matrix X, which is 2 by 3, using the J function. We then pass that matrix to the RANDGEN subroutine as its first argument and fill every element of that matrix with simulated values by specifying the distribution name, Normal, and its parameters, 10 and 2. This has a very similar syntax to the RAND function that we learned about in Chapter 4.

There are lots of different distributions that you can use with the RANDGEN subroutine. Table 7.5 lists the univariate probability distributions, and of course, you want to check the online documentation to make sure you know how to use the parameters, what order they should be in, and to see the multivariate distributions as well.

Table 7.5: Univariate Distributions

| Bernoulli | Beta | Binomial |
|---|---|---|
| Cauchy | Chi-Square | Erlang |
| Exponential | F | Gamma |
| Geometric | Hypergeometric | Laplace |
| Logistic | Lognormal | Negative Binomial |
| Normal | Normal Mixture | Pareto |
| Poisson | T | Table |
| Triangle | Tweedie | Uniform |
| Wald | Weibull | |

RANDFUN Function

If you want to vectorize your code, just like you would in R, for example, using RNORM, you can use the RANDFUN function to simulate random vectors using the following syntax:

*result* = **RANDFUN**(*n, dist-name<,parm1><,parm2><,parm3>*);

In Program 7.8, we want a vector that is 10 by 1, so we pass it the argument 10, and the same arguments as before on the RANDGEN subroutine (the distribution name and its parameters).

**Program 7.8: RANDFUN function**
```
X = randfun(10,"Normal",10,2);
```

Notice that because this is a function, we have to use an assignment statement with the RANDFUN function, unlike the RANDGEN module, which is a subroutine.

**Tip:** Inside loops, it is more efficient to use the RANDGEN subroutine.

## Common IML Modules

In this section, we will discuss some other useful modules that you might want to be aware of. Most modules are intuitive and identical to R. For example, the ABS() function returns the absolute value for each element in a matrix and is identical to R syntax. EXPonentiate, LOG, SQuare RooT, MAX, MIN, PROD, and SUM all operate the exact same way as R. Table 7.6 lists some useful modules to know.

Table 7.6: IML Modules

| Mathematical | ABS, EXP, LOG, SQRT |
|---|---|
| Reduction | MAX, MIN, PROD, SUM |
| Matrix Inquiry | ALL, ANY, LOC, COUNTN |
| Matrix Reshaping | VECDIAG, REPEAT, SHAPE |
| Random Number Generation | CALL RANDGEN, CALL RANDSEED |
| Statistical | CORR, COV, MEAN, CALL QNTL |
| Numerical Analysis | CALL SPLINE, BSPLINE |
| Linear Algebra | DET, TRACE, INV, CALL EIGEN, SOLVE, CALL SVD, CALL QR, ROOT |
| Optimization | CALL NLPNRA |
| ... | ... |

You should see some familiar modules in Table 7.6. We have already talked about random number generation, some statistical functions, and how find the correlation and covariance. You can use the MEAN function (the same as colMeans in R), which takes the mean of each column of your matrix. You can find any quantile that you want using the QNTL subroutine.

You can do some numerical analysis with splines, lots of modules for linear algebra like the DETerminant, TRACE, INVerse, the Eigen subroutine, and solve a linear system of equations. You can do QR decomposition or the Cholesky root. And there are lots and lots of optimization subroutines as well, with many more listed in the documentation.

## Matrix Reshaping

### REPEAT Function

This section covers some very simple but useful modules. The REPEAT function is similar to RET function in R, and uses the following syntax:

*result* = **REPEAT**(*matrix, nrow, ncol*);

or

*result* = **REPEAT**(*matrix, freq*);

In the following code, we have a matrix X, which is 2 by 2. We create a new matrix Y using the first form of the REPEAT function, and are repeating X as if it were a 2-by-2 matrix.

```
Y = repeat (X,2,2);
```

$$X = \begin{bmatrix} 1 & 2 \\ 3 & 4 \end{bmatrix} \quad Y = \begin{bmatrix} 1 & 2 & 1 & 2 \\ 3 & 4 & 3 & 4 \\ 1 & 2 & 1 & 2 \\ 3 & 4 & 3 & 4 \end{bmatrix}$$

The first form of the REPEAT function creates a new matrix by repeating the values of matrix nrow times across the rows and ncol times across the columns. Repeating that matrix gives us the 4-by-4 matrix. Notice each 2-by-2 cell is the same X matrix.

Likewise, we can repeat each element of the matrix using the alternative syntax. The second form of the REPEAT function returns a row vector with each value in matrix repeated the number of times specified in freq.

```
Y = repeat (X, {2 2 3 3});
```

$$X = \begin{bmatrix} 1 & 2 \\ 3 & 4 \end{bmatrix} \quad Y = \begin{bmatrix} 1 & 1 & 2 & 2 & 3 & 3 & 3 & 4 & 4 & 4 \end{bmatrix}$$

Here we are repeating the first element two times, the second element two times, the third and fourth element three times each, and that simply returns a row vector.

If you are working with character data in IML and you need to concatenate vectors, you are going to use the CONCAT function using the following syntax:

*result* = **CONCAT**(*matrix1*, *matrix2*,...);

This function is helpful when you are creating column or row headers. Program 7.9 shows an example of using the CONCAT function.

**Program 7.9: CONCAT Function**
```
pre = j(1,3,"data");
post = char(1:3);
result = concat(pre,post);
```

In the first line of Program 7.9, we create a vector, pre, which is a 1-by-3 vector where every element is the word, data. Then we use the sequence 1 to 3, using the CHAR function to say it is character data. Finally, we concatenate these two character vectors, pre and post. The result is the following vector, which can be used a column or row header:

$$result = \begin{bmatrix} data\ 1 & data\ 2 & data\ 3 \end{bmatrix}$$

## Matrix Inquiry

Matrix inquiry functions are extremely useful when you are doing conditional processing. We will look at five matrix inquiry functions: ANY(), ALL(), ISEMPTY(), SAMPLE(), and UNIQUE(). Let's look at how the first three functions work using the 2 by 2 matrix X.

$$X = \begin{bmatrix} 1 & 2 \\ 3 & 4 \end{bmatrix}$$

### ANY Function

The ANY function says, "Is any element in X greater than 3?" using the following syntax:

```
A = any(X>3);  →  A=1
```

Because it's true that there is an element in matrix X that is greater than 3, it returns the binary result 1.

### ALL Function

Are all elements of the matrix X greater than 3?

```
B = all(X>3);  →  B=0
```

No, all elements of matrix X are not greater than 3, so it returns the element 0.

### ISEMPTY Function

The ISEMPTY function checks to see whether a matrix is empty, that is, if it has no rows or columns.

```
c = isempty(X);  →  C=0
```

Of course, we have already made X, so it's not empty. Therefore, it returns a value of 0.

### SAMPLE and UNIQUE Functions

The SAMPLE and UNIQUE functions are identical to R. They use the following syntax:

*result*= **SAMPLE**(*matrix, n, <method>,<prob>*);

*result*= **UNIQUE**(*matrix*);

The SAMPLE function generates a random sample of the elements of the matrix. The SAMPLE function method can be "REPLACE", "NOREPLACE", or "WOR". The method of "WOR" specifies a simple random sampling without replacement. After the elements are randomly selected, their order is randomly permuted. The prob argument is a vector with the same number of elements as the matrix. The vector specifies the sampling probability for the elements of the matrix. The SAMPLE function scales the elements of prob so that they do not need to sum to 1.

The UNIQUE function returns a row vector with the sorted set of all elements in the matrix without duplicates. The matrix can be either numeric or character.

The COUNTUNIQUE function returns the number of unique values in a matrix, or the length of the returned matrix from the UNIQUE function.

## Linear Algebra Modules

Table 7.7 shows the general form of some useful linear algebra modules in SAS. There are many more modules available on the documentation page.

**Table 7.7: Linear Algebra Modules**

| INV(X) | Computes the inverse of a square nonsingular matrix. |
|---|---|
| SOLVE(A,B) | Solves a system of linear equations. |
| ROOT(X) | Performs the Cholesky decomposition of a symmetric positive definite matrix. |
| GINV(X) | Computes the Moore-Penrose generalized inverse of a matrix. |
| SVD(X) | Computes the singular value decomposition of a matrix. |

You can use the INV for inverse and SOLVE to solve a linear system of equations the same way as in R. For example, you can just replace the inverse of x transpose x with the INV function, as opposed to doing the singular value decomposition if you wanted.

The SAS documentation lists all the IML functions and subroutines. Another great resource is the SAS/IML blog at blogs.sas.com/content/iml. Finally, if you are not too comfortable with IML or simply matrix language operations in general, another helpful resource is the book *Statistical Programming with SAS/IML® Software* by Rick Wicklin.

## Create a Module

SAS is not going to have all the built-in modules that you're going to want to use, so now you'll learn how to create your own modules to implement analyses from a journal article or implement a proprietary algorithm developed at your company. Creating a module can assist in creating any type of IML script.

A module always begins with the START statement and ends with the FINISH statement. The START statement instructs IML to enter a module-collect mode. In this mode, IML gathers the statements of a module rather than executing them immediately. The FINISH statement signals the end of a module, as shown in the following syntax:

**START** *name <(argument1, argument2,...)>*
  **<GLOBAL**(*argument1, argument2,...*)>;
  *statements*;
  **<RETURN**(*matrix*);>
**FINISH**;

*Name* is the user-defined module name. *Arguments* are input or output matrices (or both) that are used or created by the module.

### Create a Function Module

Let's first create a SAS function module. Remember, function modules return only a single matrix. They require the RETURN statement and are executed using an ASSIGNMENT statement. Program 7.10 is an example of a function module.

**Program 7.10: Function Module**
```
start add(a,b);
    c = a + b;
    return(c);
finish;

x = {1 2, 3 4};
y = {5 6, 7 8};
z = add(x,y);
```

In Program 7.10, we start with the START statement and create a new function called ADD. We have two arguments, a and b. Inside the module creation, we create a new variable, c, which is equal to a plus b, and because this is a function, we have to use the RETURN statement, so we are returning c, and then finishing with the FINISH statement.

Recall that in R, all matrices outside of the function are global but are also pulled into the local symbol table. For example, in R as shown in Figure 7.3, we have a function called ADD with one argument, a, and you will notice we are adding a to the variable y. This was created outside the function, but R automatically pulls it into the function and uses it.

**Figure 7.3: R Script**

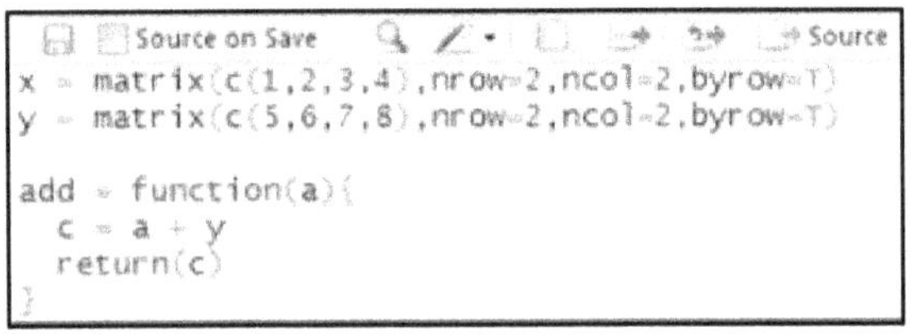

To do the same thing in SAS, we just have to use the GLOBAL option in the START statement. The GLOBAL clause is used to specify variables that are used in the module but not specified as inputs. In Program 7.11, we have two matrices in IML, x and y, which are both 2 by 2. We create a new matrix z, set that equal to the new ADD function, and specify the arguments x and y. Then we have access to use the z matrix.

**Program 7.11: GLOBAL Option**
```
x = {1 2, 3 4};
y = {5 6, 7 8};
```

```
start add(a) global(y);
    c = a + y;
    return(c);
finish;


z = add(x);
```

In Program 7.10, we are creating the ADD function, but only one argument, a. We are pulling y into the local symbol table, and have c equal to a plus y, returning that new variable c.


### Create a Subroutine Module

Subroutine modules are used to output multiple matrices. This is similar to returning a list in R. The symbols X, Y, A, and B are local symbols, meaning that they are not recognized outside of the user-defined module. As a result, you can specify any symbol as the output matrices in the CALL statement.

If you create a module without any arguments, all the matrices defined outside the creation of the module are pulled into the local symbol table. In Program 7.12, we create x and y. We have module ADD with no arguments, and are adding x plus y, which was defined outside the module c. Notice that this is the first instance of a subroutine, so we are executing it with a CALL statement, and don't have the RETURN statement.

**Program 7.12: Subroutine Module**
```
x = {1 2, 3 4};
y = {5 6, 7 8};

start add;
    c = x + y;
finish;

call add;
```

Recall that subroutine modules do not return a matrix. They create matrices—a very subtle distinction, but important for the programming. When you are creating a subroutine, you do not use the RETURN statement, nor do you use an ASSIGNMENT statement to call it. You use the CALL or the RUN statement.

Program 7.13 shows an earlier subroutine that we covered, the EIGEN subroutine. We have a 2-by-2 matrix and are using the EIGEN subroutine in the CALL statement. We are passing it one argument, x, and creating two matrices, evals and evecs, which represent the eigenvalue decomposition. Then we will have access to actually use them.

**Program 7.13: Eigen Subroutine**
```
x = {1 2,3 4};
call eigen(evals,evecs,x);
print evals evecs;
```

Remember that if you want more than one matrix, you can return only one in a function, but you can create several in a subroutine. In Program 7.14, we will create the subroutine called ADDSUB. The output matrices are on the left of the arguments, x and y, and then the input matrices are on the right, a and b. It's completely fine to mismatch these, but it is the syntax used on the online doc page, so you might want to use the same syntax to avoid any confusion.

**Program 7.14: ADDSUB Subroutine**
```
start addsub(x,y,a,b);
    x = a + b;
    y = a - b;
finish;
```

```
matOne = {1 2, 3 4};
matTwo = {5 6, 7 8};

call addsub(add,sub,matOne,matTwo);
```

Notice that the output matrices have to be the same exact name as the matrices inside the module, so x corresponds to x and y corresponds to y. After you call the subroutine, then you can change the created matrices' names. We are creating ADD and SUB and passing in the arguments matOne and matTwo, which are both 2-by-2 matrices.

## Storage Techniques

Just like we save SAS data sets on disk, we can also save modules and matrices on disk for later retrieval. We can store and reload IML modules and matrices, save work for a later session, and conserve memory by saving large intermediate results for later use.

SAS/IML storage catalogs are specially structured SAS files that are located in a SAS library. A SAS/IML catalog contains entries that are either matrices or modules. Like other SAS files, SAS/IML catalogs have two-level names in the form libref.catalog. The first-level name, libref, is a name assigned to the SAS library to which the catalog belongs. The second-level name, catalog, is the name of the catalog file.

When you store a matrix, IML automatically stores the matrix name, its type, its dimension, and its current values. Modules are stored in the form of their compiled code. After modules are loaded, they do not need to be parsed again, making their use very efficient.

The default libref is initially **work**, and the default catalog is **imlstor**. Thus, the default storage catalog is called **work.imlstor**. You can change the storage catalog (or both the library reference and catalog) with the RESET STORAGE command. You can list all modules and matrices in the current storage catalog using the SHOW STORAGE command.

To create a new catalog to save modules or matrices, use the RESET STORAGE statement. Set that statement equal to a library (work or another library), followed by a period and then the catalog name using the following syntax:

RESET STORAGE = <libref.>catalog;

This statement saves everything in a catalog as specially structured SAS files, located in your SAS library.

You can also use the RESET STORAGE statement to tell SAS what existing catalog you are pointing to. After you create a catalog and you want to load a matrix back into IML, run the same RESET STORAGE statement. The name RESET is a bit unfortunate in that regard because it's not actually resetting anything in that instance.

If you want to see everything in your catalog, you can just run the SHOW STORAGE statement on its own line as follows:

SHOW STORAGE;

### Catalog Management Statements

In addition to the RESET STORAGE and SHOW STORAGE catalog managements, Table 7.8 shows three additional keywords that you should know—LOAD, REMOVE, and STORE.

**Table 7.8: Catalog Management Keywords**

| Keyword | Description |
| --- | --- |
| LOAD | recalls entries back into the IML workspace. |

| Keyword | Description |
|---|---|
| REMOVE | deletes entries from the catalog. |
| STORE | places IML modules, matrices, or both into catalog storage |

For example, if you are working with the STORE keyword, you can say STORE and then list your matrices. You can also say STORE, specify the keyword MODULE, set that equal to in parentheses a list of modules, or you can do both. You can say STORE MODULE equal to, list the modules, and then after, specify the matrices.

Notice the following:

- A statement with no operands acts on all modules and matrices.
- The special operand _ALL_ can be used to specify all modules, all matrices, or all modules *and* matrices.
- If only one module is specified, then the parentheses around the module name are not required.

Table 7.9 shows a few more specific examples of how to use statements.

**Table 7.9: STORE Statement Examples**

| Statement | Description |
|---|---|
| `reset storage=sp4r.cat1;` | Specifies the storage catalog to be in libref **sp4r** with the catalog name **cat1** |
| `store expense;` | Saves the matrix **EXPENSE** onto disk, in **sp4r.cat1** |
| `store module=impute;` | Saves the user-defined module IMPUTE in **sp4r.cat1** |
| `store module=_all_;` | Saves all modules in the current IML session in **sp4r.cat1** |
| `store module=(impute) x y;` | Saves the module IMPUTE and the matrices **x** and **y** in **sp4r.cat1** |
| `store;` | Saves all matrices and modules in the current IML session in **sp4r.cat1**. This can help you save your complete IML environment before exiting an IML session. Then you can use the LOAD statement in a subsequent session to restore the environment and resume your work. |
| `load;` | Can be used to restore matrices and modules from storage back into the IML active workspace |
| `remove;` | Can be used to remove modules or matrices that are no longer needed from the catalog. The REMOVE command has the same form as the STORE command and the LOAD command. |

> **Tip:** The keyword STORE can be replaced with either LOAD or REMOVE, and the syntax still holds.

Remember that IML is in RAM. SAS data sets are on disk. You need to be a little bit more conscious of how much memory you are using in IML. Here are a few tips to reduce memory use for computers that have less than 8GB of RAM:

- Use the FREE statement to free matrices that are no longer needed.
- Use the STORE statement to store matrices on disk and then use the FREE statement to free their values. Restore the matrices later using the LOAD statement.
- Reformulate your approach to use smaller matrices (for example, by using VAR and WHERE clauses where applicable).

The FREE statement frees matrix storage spaces to make room for more data (matrices) in the workspace. The FREE statement is used mostly in large applications or under tight memory constraints using the following syntax:

**FREE** *matrices*;

**FREE** / *<matrices>*;

The FREE statements are very easy to use. If you wanted to get rid of the matrices x and y, you would say the following:

```
FREE X Y;
```

If you wanted to free all the matrices in your IML workspace, use the forward slash:

```
Free /;
```

If you want to free everything except matrix a and b, just list those matrices after the forward slash like so:

```
FREE / A B;
```

Notice that the STORE statement stores only matrices and modules. It does not free them from memory, so you can still reference them later in the same IML session. If you also issued the FREE statement afterward, the matrices are no longer in the memory, and you must use the LOAD statement to restore them.

## Call SAS Data Sets and Procedures

In this section, you will learn how to create a matrix using a SAS data set, export a matrix to a SAS data set, or add data to an existing SAS data set by stacking it underneath. First, we have to talk about Open data sets. An Open data set is one that is ready for Read or Write access or both. You can use one of the following three statements to open a data set:

- **USE** enables Read access. That lets us open our SAS data set and read values into an IML matrix.
- **EDIT** enables Read and Write access to an existing data set.
- **CREATE** gives both Read and Write access. It simply creates a new data set.

Regardless of which of these three statements you use, you want to use the CLOSE statement immediately following it. That will simply close the Open data set. If you do not close, you might not have access to either use it or open it with your mouse. If you forget to use the CLOSE statement, SAS closes the open data set when you exit SAS/IML with the QUIT statement.

If you open a data set with the USE statement, you can still open the data set manually to view the table. However, opening a data set with the EDIT statement does not permit you to open and view the data table manually.

## Create a Matrix Using a SAS Data Set

To create a matrix using a SAS data set, we will use the USE, READ, and CLOSE statements. Program 7.15 uses a data set called CLASS. We read in the data with the READ statement and close the Open data set with the CLOSE statement.

**Program 7.15: Create a Matrix using Class Data Set**

```
use class;
read all var {height weight}
    where (sex='M') into imlClass;
close class;
```

Let's talk more about the READ statement. This is where all the action happens. There are lots of different options, as you can see in the following syntax:

**READ** *<range>* **<VAR** *operand>* **<WHERE***(expression)>*
      **<INTO** *name* **<[ROWNAME=***row-name* **COLNAME=***col-name]>>*;

In Program 7.15, we want to read in a specified range, read in all observations, and only read in the variables with the VAR option. We give it a character vector and read in only the variables height and weight from that CLASS data set. Then we use a WHERE option to read in observations conditionally where sex is equal to M. Finally, we use the keyword INTO to throw all of that data into a new matrix called IMLClass. You can also use ROWNAME and COLNAME options to create new ROWNAME and COLNAMES to be printed using the PRINT statement in IML.

## Save a Matrix as a SAS Data Set

If you have a matrix that you want to save as a SAS data set, we will use the CREATE statement to do that. If you want to add data to an existing SAS data set, we will use the EDIT statement.

### CREATE Statement

There are two forms of the CREATE statement, depending on the data you are writing to a SAS data set. The first form uses the following syntax:

**CREATE** *SAS-data-set* **<VAR** *{operand}>*;

We run the CREATE statement and specify the new SAS data set we are creating. And if we are writing vectors to the new SAS data set, use the VAR option and specify the names of the vectors as a row vector. The good thing about this option is that the names of the vectors will be used as the SAS data set variable names. If the VAR option is not used, a variable is created for every SAS/IML matrix that is in scope,and the matrix names are used as variable names in the new data set.

Each matrix used to create the data set corresponds to a single variable in the data set. If a matrix with multiple rows and multiple columns is used as a data set variable, its contents are written to the data set in row-major order.

The second form of the CREATE statement appends a matrix to a SAS data set, using the following syntax:

**CREATE** *SAS-data-set* **FROM** *matrix-name*
      **<[ROWNAME=***row-name*
        **COLNAME=***column-name]>*;

When the FROM keyword is used in the CREATE statement, each column in the source matrix is treated as a distinct variable in the newly created data set. As a best practice, you should use the COLNAME option. That will let you set the SAS data set variable names directly in the CREATE statement. This way, you don't have to use a DATA step to change the names. Why? Because if you append a matrix to a data set, the default names will be col1, col2, col3, and so on.

### APPEND Statement

The CREATE statement opens a data set only for input or output. You need to use the APPEND statement to write to the data set.

There are three different forms of the APPEND statement, but they depend on the CREATE statement that you are using. Let's look at the syntax of the three different forms below:

**APPEND;**

**APPEND VAR** *matrix-list*;

**APPEND FROM** *append_matrix* <[**ROWNAME**=*row-name*]>;

To create a SAS data set using an IML matrix, use the statements CREATE, APPEND, and CLOSE. Here is an example of creating a SAS data set using the first form of the APPEND Statement:

```
create data1 var{name age};
append;
close data1;
```

In the example above, we are creating a new data set called data1, and writing two vectors to that data set with a VAR option, name and age. Then we have to explicitly tell SAS to append that data with the APPEND statement, and finally, close the open data set.

The VAR option can be used in either the CREATE statement or the APPEND statement but not both. The VAR option specifies which vectors to pass to a SAS data set. The VAR option is not used to pass a matrix to a SAS data set. Here is an example of the APPEND statement using the VAR option:

```
create data2;
append var{name age};
close data2;
```

The only difference from the previous example is that we have brought the VAR option down into the APPEND statement.

In the third example, we are creating a new data set called data3 from a matrix called matrix3. To change the SAS data set variable names right in the CREATE statement, use the COLNAME option as shown below:

```
create data3 from matrix3[colname={week1, week2, week3, week4}];
append from matrix3;
close data3;
```

Set the COLNAME option equal to a vector of the variable names week1 through week4. Use the APPEND FROM statement to append a matrix and list the same matrix from the CREATE statement. Again, close the open data set.

### EDIT Statement

If a data set already exists, you can open the data set with the EDIT statement, add data, and then close the data set as shown in the following example:

```
edit data2;
append from matrix4;
close data2;
```

In the example, we are editing the SAS data set, data2, and using the APPEND FROM statement to stack the matrix4 matrix underneath the existing SAS data set. The important thing to remember is that the matrix has to have the same number of columns as the existing SAS data set.

## Call SAS Procedures

Now that we know how to put matrices into a SAS data set, how do we run procedures on those SAS data sets without exiting IML? Remember, once we exit IML, everything in that workspace that is not saved is deleted.

Here are a few benefits of calling SAS procedures directly from IML:

- You can call SAS procedures without exiting IML.
- SAS procedures can be used within IML modules.
- Matrix values can be used as parameters for SAS procedures.
- You can execute SAS procedures conditionally or within loops.

To call SAS procedures from IML, we will use the SUBMIT and ENDSUBMIT statements. In the SUBMIT statement, we can pass it parameters, specifically, matrices that are in IML. And then we can refer to those matrices as arguments with the following syntax:

**SUBMIT** *<parameters>* / *<options>*;
*statements*;
**ENDSUBMIT**;

The statements between the SUBMIT and ENDSUBMIT statements are referred to as a SUBMIT block. The parameters value specifies one or more option matrices whose values are substituted into language statements in the SUBMIT block. SUBMIT blocks can contain the following:

- SAS procedures
- DATA steps
- ODS commands
- Other SAS statements

A SUBMIT block executes only after the ENDSUBMIT; line is run.

## Statistical Graphics in SAS/IML

In R, when we generate data, we can plot it with a PLOT function. In SAS/IML, we cannot directly plot data. We have to export that matrix to a SAS data set and then run the SGPLOT procedure to create a graphic.

SAS/IML provides subroutines that enable you to create statistical graphics. The following subroutines use the SUBMIT and ENDBUSMIT statements to call PROC SGPLOT:

- BAR call
- BOX call
- HISTOGRAM call
- SERIES call
- HEATMAPCONT call
- HEATMAPDISC call

This is going to create a new SAS data set, and then pass that data set to the SGPLOT procedure. All you have to do is use the single subroutine. Go to the following web page to see an overview of statistical graphics in SAS/IML:

http://support.sas.com/documentation/cdl/en/imlug/68150/HTML/default/viewer.htm#imlug_graphics_sect 001.htm.

Let's look at an example using the SCATTER subroutine. Imagine we have read the Cars data set into IML and we want to quickly create a scatter plot directly in IML. We will use the SCATTER subroutine s shown in Program 7.16.

**Program 7.16: SCATTER Subroutine**

```
title "Scatter Plot with Default Properties";
call Scatter(MPG_City, MPG_Highway)
label={"MPG_City" "MPG_Highway"};
```

**Output 7.16: Results of Program 7.16**

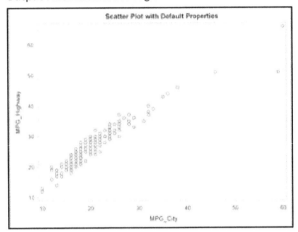

In Program 7.16, we assign MPG_City as the x-axis variable and MPG_Highway as the y-axis variable. Notice that we are also passing the subroutine the label and title option. You can pass the subroutine whatever options that you would use in the SGPLOT procedure. It creates a SAS data set behind the scenes and then uses SGPLOT to create the graphic shown in Output 7.16. You can use whatever SGPLOT options you want directly in the IML subroutine, all of which can be found in the documentation.

# Simulations

In this section, we want to use Monte Carlo Simulation and SAS/IML to do the following—obtain an approximate solution to a problem or evaluate statistic methods. By the end of this section, you should be able to create your own function or subroutine and then use it inside a simulation in some type of loop and save the data for each iteration then analyze all the data you have saved.

## Conditional Processing Syntax

### IF, ELSE IF, and ELSE Statements

The good thing about the IML simulations is that we already have all the syntax requirements. Recall that we can use IF, ELSE IF, and ELSE statements directly in IML using the following syntax:

**IF** *expression* **THEN** *statement*;
**<ELSE IF** *expression* **THEN** *statement*;>
**<ELSE** *statement*;>

In Program 7.16, we use conditional processing statements in IML that are identical to the statements used in a DATA step. As in a DATA step, the ELSE IF and ELSE statements are completely optional for conditional processing. In addition, the user can specify multiple ELSE IF statements.

**Program 7.17: Conditional Processing**

```
X = {1 2, 3 4};
miss = loc(x=.);
flag = isempty(miss);

if flag=0 then print x;
else print "empty matrix!";
```

In Program 7.17, we are saying that if the matrix flag is equal to zero, then print x. Otherwise, the catchall ELSE statement prints the empty matrix.

## DO Loops

The DO loop will be our main tool for doing simulation. To execute multiple statements conditionally, use a DO statement with the following syntax:

**DO;**
  *statements*;
**END;**

The DO statement specifies that the statements following the DO statement are executed as a group until a matching END statement appears. DO statements often appear with clauses invoking iterative execution or in IF-THEN/ELSE statements so that the group of statements is executed only when the IF condition is satisfied.

The DO loop in IML is identical to the FOR loop in R. In Program 7.18, DO i equals 1 to 10 with the specified increment of 1. Then we print i every iteration, and use the END statement to end the DO group.

**Program 7.18: DO Loop**
```
do i=1 to 10 by 1;
print i;
end;
```

Remember when we talked about the DO loop in Chapter 4, we said use an OUTPUT statement to write all the data from those iterations to a data set? In IML and in a simulation, we are not going to use the OUTPUT statement. You will have to tell SAS explicitly what data from the iteration you want to save, just like in R.

## SUBMIT Blocks with Loops and Conditions

SUBMIT blocks can be combined with IF statements to execute SAS procedures and DATA steps conditionally. SUBMIT blocks can be combined with loops to execute SAS procedures and DATA steps repeatedly.

Let's look at an example in Program 7.19.

**Program 7.19: SUBMIT Block**
```
proc iml;
    do i = 1 to 1000;
        if i <= 500 then do;
            submit block;
        end;
        else do;
            submit block;
        end;
    end;
quit;
```

In Program 7.19, do i equals 1 to 1,000. If i is less than or equal to 500, then do the following— execute multiple statements. Otherwise, when the iteration value is 501 or greater, do something else. So we simply combine all these ideas for a simulation.

## DO WHILE Loops

A DO WHILE statement duplicates the **while()** function in R using the following syntax:

**DO WHILE**(*expression*);
  *statements*;
**END;**

In Program 7.20, we pass the DO WHILE statement an expression. While x is less than 5, we want to print x. Don't forget to increment your expression-- x is equal to x plus 1. This way, it actually turns off eventually. Don't forget your END statement.

**Program 7.20: DO WHILE Loop**

```
x=1;
do while(x<5);
    print x;
    x = x+1;
end;
```

## Example: Monty Hall Problem

Let's do a fun simulation with an example that you are probably familiar with: the Monty Hall problem. You are a guest on a game show, and the host presents you with three doors. One door hides a car; the other two doors hide goats.

The host asks you to pick a door. You pick door number 1. The host, who knows what is behind each door, opens one of the two doors that you did not pick and always reveals a goat. The host will never show you the car. Then, the host gives you the option of staying with your initial choice or switching to the remaining closed door. What should you do, stay or switch?

If we were to solve this problem analytically, we would find that switching yields a 2/3 chance of winning the car and staying with the initial choice yields a 1/3 chance of winning a car. But maybe we don't want to solve the analytical method, or maybe we are working on a much harder problem, so let's do a simulation to find an empirical result for this problem.

> **Tip**: Make your simulations more efficient by removing DO loops when possible.

1. Let the number of simulations be 10,000 and set the random number seed to 802.

   ```
   proc iml;
       numberIterations=10000;
        call randseed(802);
   ```

2. Start the simulation loop, which runs the number of times equal to **numberIterations**. The first step in simulating the Monty Hall problem is to choose which of the three doors hides the car. Use the SAMPLE function to draw a random door, {1 2 3}.

   ```
   *Begin simulation;
   do iteration=1 to numberIterations;
       doors = {1 2 3};
       carDoor=sample(doors,1);
   ```

3. For the sake of simplicity, always choose door 1. Monty Hall never opens the chosen door and never opens the door hiding the car. If the chosen door (door 1) hides the car, Monty randomly chooses between doors 2 and 3 (represented by a draw from a Bernoulli distribution with probability .5). If the car is hidden behind door 2, Monty Hall must open door 3. (He cannot open the door hiding the car or the door that you chose). If the car is hidden behind door 3, Monty Hall must open door 2.

   ```
   *Pick door for Monty Hall to open;
   if carDoor=1 then openDoor=randfun(1,"Bernoulli",.5) + 2;
   else if carDoor=2 then openDoor=3;
   else if carDoor=3 then openDoor=2;
   ```

4. Using a switching strategy requires switching to the unopened door that was not previously chosen. If Monty Hall opened door 2, switch to door 3. If Monty Hall opened door 3, switch to door 2.

```
*Determine door for switching strategy;
if openDoor=2 then switchDoor=3;
else if openDoor=3 then switchDoor=2;
```

5. If the car is behind door number 1, then the staying strategy wins because door number 1 was initially chosen. If the car is behind the door that would be chosen based on the switching strategy, then the switching strategy wins.

```
*Determine which strategy wins;
if carDoor=1 then stayWin=1;
else stayWin=0;
if carDoor=switchDoor then switchWin=1;
else switchWin=0;
/*switchWin=carDoor=switchDoor;*/
```

6. Append the results for the current iteration to a matrix called **results** and end the simulation loop.

```
*Collect results to a single matrix;
results=results // (iteration || carDoor || openDoor || stayWin
    || switchWin);
end;
```

7. Print the first 10 rows of the **results** matrix to show the outcome for every iteration. Calculate and print the percentage of iterations for which each strategy won.

```
reset noname;
resultsSubset = results[1:10,];
print resultsSubset [colname={iteration carDoor openDoor
    stayWin switchWin}];
percentageWins=results[:,{4 5}];
print percentageWins [colname={stay switch}
```

| ITERATION | CARDOOR | OPENDOOR | STAYWIN | SWITCHWIN |
|---|---|---|---|---|
| 1 | 2 | 3 | 0 | 1 |
| 2 | 3 | 2 | 0 | 1 |
| 3 | 2 | 3 | 0 | 1 |
| 4 | 1 | 3 | 1 | 0 |
| 5 | 1 | 2 | 1 | 0 |
| 6 | 2 | 3 | 0 | 1 |
| 7 | 2 | 3 | 0 | 1 |
| 8 | 3 | 2 | 0 | 1 |
| 9 | 2 | 3 | 0 | 1 |
| 10 | 2 | 3 | 0 | 1 |

| STAY | SWITCH |
|---|---|
| 0.3297 | 0.6703 |

## IML Simulations

There are three simulation methods in IML.

1.  The first method is to simulate entirely in IML and ignore SAS procedures. Just code everything yourself.

2.  The second method is to iteratively call SAS procedures. This is most similar to using R functions in your simulation, but it is the most inefficient method in SAS.

3.  Finally, you can use a SAS procedure and a BY statement to avoid any type of looping. That tells SAS to analyze each data set independently. First output all simulated data to a single SAS data set with a variable indicating the iteration number. Analyze the data using a SAS procedure (for example, PROC GLM) with a BY statement, and output the results to a SAS data set. Separate results are output for each iteration.

Analyzing each simulated data set one at a time is very inefficient. If you have to use a SAS procedure, the third method is the most efficient method.

For example, if each SAS data set is 20 observations, and you are doing 1,000 simulations, you want to output all 20,000 observations, and an index variable specifying which observation comes from which data set. The first 20 observations should have a variable indicating the number one. The second 20 should have a variable indicating the number two, and so on. Then, you pass all this data to a single procedure like PROC GLM and pass to the BY statement the index variable iteration number. When you do that, SAS is going to analyze each one of those data sets independently. And SAS will output the results for each data set to a single SAS data set. So separate results are output for each iteration.

# Exercises

## Multiple Choice

1. Suppose you want to print your salary for the week. Assume that you worked 40 hours and earn $9.35 per hour. Which of the following show the correct syntax for printing your salary? Keep in mind that brackets are not required to assign a scalar. Select all that apply.
   a. Y=40*9.35; Print Y;
   b. 40*9.35;
   c. Print (40*9.35);
   d. Print 40*9.35;

2. Let X be an m-by-n matrix. How would you use a SAS reduction operator to reproduce the rowMeans() and min() functions in R?
   a. X[,:] and X[><,]
   b. X[:,] and X(>:<,>:<)
   c. X{,:} and X[><,><]
   d. X[,:] and X[><,><]

3. The PROC IML code below prints the 0.75 quantile from matrix X.

   ```
   Q = call qntl(X,{0.75});
   print Q;
   ```

   a. True
   b. False

4. Which of the following statements about SAS modules are true? Select all that apply.
   a. Modules are defined by START and FINISH keywords.
   b. Functions use the RETURN statement
   c. The RETURN statement can handle multiple arguments.
   d. Subroutines can be executed by the CALL statement.

5. How do you recall the module rock and the matrix pony into a new SAS/IML session from the mycat catalog in the Work directory?
   a. RESET STORAGE; LOAD module=(rock) pony;
   b. RESET STORAGE=mycat; LOAD module=(rock) pony;
   c. STORAGE=mycat; LOAD module=(rock) pony;
   d. RESET STORAGE=mycat; LOAD rock pony;

6. Which statements are true regarding importing SAS data sets and exporting IML matrices? Select all that apply.
   a. The statements USE, READ, and CLOSE are used to pass a SAS data set into IML.
   b. The statements CREATE, APPEND, and CLOSE are used to pass an IML matrix to a SAS data set.
   c. Names of IML vectors are passed to the SAS data set as variable names.
   d. The user must specify the column names when creating a SAS data set from an IML matrix.

## Short Answer

1. Navigate to the SAS/IML documentation and peruse the statements, functions, and subroutines. Choose a few that look familiar to you and see what they do. Next, find the LOC function and see what it does.

1. **Practicing with Basic Operations**

   In this exercise, you perform operations on the data used in the previous demonstration. Use the code below at the beginning of the exercise program.

   ```
   proc iml;
   items =        {'Groceries','Utilities','Rent','Car Expenses',
                   'Fun Money','Personal Expenses'};
   weeks =        {'Week 1','Week 2','Week 3','Week 4'};
   amounts =      { 96  78  82   93,
                    61  77  62   68,
                   300 300 300 300,
                    25  27  98   18,
                    55  34  16   53,
                   110  85  96 118};
   weeklyIncome ={900 850 1050 950};
   weeklyExpenses=amounts[+,];
   ```

   a. Create a 1 x 4 matrix named **proportionIncomeSpent** whose elements are the proportion of each week's income that went to expenses. Use the RESET statement to suppress the automatic printing of matrix names. Print the **proportionIncomeSpent** matrix with the values of **weeks** used as column labels and PERCENT7.2 used as a format.

      PROC IML Output

      ```
      Proportion of income spent each week

        Week 1   Week 2   Week 3   Week 4

        71.9%    70.7%    62.3%    68.4%
      ```

   b. Create a 1 x 4 matrix named **proportionIncomeSaved** whose elements are equal to the proportion of each week's income that did not go to expenses. That is, use an implicit loop to subtract the values of **proportionIncomeSpent** from one. Print the **proportionIncomeSaved** matrix with the values of weeks used as column labels and PERCENT7.2 used as a format.

      PROC IML Output

      ```
      Proportion of income saved each week

        Week 1   Week 2   Week 3   Week 4

        28.1%    29.3%    37.7%    31.6%
      ```

   c. Create a 6 x 4 matrix named **proportionSpentPerItem** whose elements are the proportion of each week's income spent on each item, by week. That is, use an implicit loop to divide the **amounts** matrix by the **weeklyIncome** matrix. Print the **proportionSpentPerItem** matrix with the values of **items** used as row labels, the values of **weeks** used as column labels, and PERCENT7.2 used as a format.

      ```
      Percentage of income spent on each item, by week
                          Week 1  Week 2  Week 3  Week 4

      Groceries           10.7%   9.18%   7.81%   9.79%
      Utilities           6.78%   9.06%   5.90%   7.16%
      Rent                33.3%   35.3%   28.6%   31.6%
      Car Expenses        2.78%   3.18%   9.33%   1.89%
      Fun Money           6.11%   4.00%   1.52%   5.58%
      Personal Expenses   12.2%   10.0%   9.14%   12.4%
      ```

d. Create a matrix named **weeklyExpenseChange** with the same number of rows as **amounts** but with one less column than **amounts** (in other words, a 6 x 3 matrix). Fill it with missing numeric values. This should be done with a matrix literal. Fill each column of **weeklyExpenseChange** with each column of **amounts** minus the previous column of **amounts**. That is, column 1 of **weeklyExpenseChange** should equal column 2 of **amounts** minus column 1 of **amounts**, and so on. Print a title and print the matrix. Use columns 2 through 4 of **weeks** as column labels and use **items** as row labels.

```
Change in spending from previous week, by item
                 Week 2      Week 3      Week 4

Groceries           -18           4          11
Utilities            16         -15           6
Rent                  0           0           0
Car Expenses          2          71         -80
Fun Money           -21         -18          37
Personal Expenses   -25          11          22
```

2. **Generating a Multiple Regression Data Matrix and Computing Parameter Estimates**

This exercise extends the ideas from the previous demonstration.

a. Generate data from a multiple regression model, $y_i = \beta_0 + \beta_1 x_{1i} + \beta_2 x_{2i} + \varepsilon_i$, with 20 samples where $\beta_0 = 3$, $\beta_1 = 2$, $\beta_2 = -1$, and $\varepsilon_i \sim N(0, \sigma = 5)$. Let $x_{1i} \sim Uniform(0, 20)$ and $x_{2i} \sim Uniform(10, 30)$. Use the seed 27606 to duplicate your results. Generate the random numbers using the RANDFUN function. Print the generated values.

| y | beta0 | beta1 | beta2 | xvals1 | xvals2 | error |
|---|---|---|---|---|---|---|
| 2.3890519 | 3 | 2 | -1 | 15.535752 | 25.086444 | -6.596008 |
| 27.055062 | | | | 19.109842 | 16.336432 | 2.1718106 |
| -4.292507 | | | | 8.7436082 | 21.76381 | -3.015913 |
| 11.835473 | | | | 12.034105 | 20.732286 | 5.4995483 |
| 18.823426 | | | | 12.89481 | 16.240074 | 6.2738806 |
| -26.1453 | | | | 1.948081 | 23.511204 | -9.530258 |
| 27.55394 | | | | 19.206666 | 15.207025 | 1.3476321 |
| 15.761662 | | | | 14.474217 | 17.647193 | 1.460422 |
| 12.815418 | | | | 12.986986 | 18.152577 | 1.9940234 |
| 19.421855 | | | | 18.214594 | 25.124106 | 5.1167724 |
| 16.696806 | | | | 15.184676 | 29.289954 | 12.617408 |
| -15.49262 | | | | 2.9719555 | 27.424333 | 2.9878057 |
| 6.7790585 | | | | 15.249747 | 20.255948 | -6.464489 |
| 31.024149 | | | | 19.654065 | 11.005698 | -0.278282 |
| 6.8295732 | | | | 9.9692864 | 27.152395 | 11.043396 |
| -8.10431 | | | | 0.0501745 | 11.999825 | 0.795166 |
| -10.70045 | | | | 1.934529 | 16.587159 | -0.982352 |
| 28.096877 | | | | 19.974169 | 10.011983 | -4.839478 |
| 5.1143731 | | | | 9.217379 | 13.189886 | -3.130499 |
| 6.3452045 | | | | 16.397849 | 27.952028 | -1.498465 |

b.  Create the design matrix and compute $\widehat{\beta} = \left( X^T X \right)^{-} X^T Y$ using the INV function. Print your results.

```
               x

1  6.9833149 28.419994
1 11.619663  13.11864
1 14.863959 25.720417
1 17.563605  14.31566
1  0.0771578 24.440131
1   16.60792 26.879481
1 14.251058 18.034902
1 14.773279 12.525219
1  1.6650986 29.064125
1 11.628301 10.744335
1   14.12347 19.860202
1  1.5470275 20.552019
1     19.547 25.236564
1 12.918223 29.589143
1  1.3057261  18.96901
1   8.558932 16.789311
1  6.7389815 20.715758
1   0.425611 20.222944
1  0.1731237 10.720545
1 13.190648 22.985184


       betaHat

     4.5097506
     2.0297133
    -1.040226
```

c.  Compute and print the estimates $\widehat{\sigma}^2$ and $\widehat{\sigma}$ where $\widehat{\sigma}^2 = \dfrac{\sum\limits_{i=1}^{n} \left( y_i - \widehat{y}_i \right)}{n-1}$. Recall that SAS does not use the ^ operator to exponentiate matrix elements.

```
sigma2Hat   sigmaHat

33.790635 5.8129713
```

3.  **Creating User-Defined Functions and Subroutines**

Standardized values are computed as $\dfrac{x - \overline{x}}{std(x)}$ where $std(x) = \sqrt{\dfrac{\sum \left( x - \overline{x} \right)}{n-1}}$ .

a.  Create a function, STANDARDIZE, that takes a matrix as an input and returns the matrix with each column standardized.

b.  Create a 10 x 3 matrix of random numbers where the first column is 123, the second column is 123, and the third column is 123. Use the seed 802 to duplicate your results. Print the matrix and then use the STANDARDIZE function to create and print the standardized matrix.

```
           mymat

11.606944 11.863687 18.710933
5.2331384 13.862579 8.2257589
5.0699716 13.325589 13.889108
9.2352147 12.471574 4.3133361
7.5553052 13.356539 1.1156816
6.7021899 12.096431 14.181072
-1.018837 14.853318 1.4487006
6.0402131 13.289878 10.497412
2.9340508 12.488342 1.2435366
11.963293 12.219451 4.9053748


           stand

 1.297565 -1.205853 1.7341685
-0.332141 0.9480863 0.0595209
-0.373861  0.369444  0.964047
 0.691142 -0.550814 -0.565355
0.2616091 0.4027946 -1.076071
0.0434776 -0.955056 1.0106784
-1.930697 2.0156739 -1.022882
-0.125782 0.3309627 0.4223396
-0.919991 -0.532745  -1.05565
1.3886794 -0.822494 -0.470797
```

c. Alter the STANDARDIZE function and create the subroutine STANDSUB. Let the subroutine take a matrix as input and output the standardized matrix, as well as the column means and standard deviations.

d. Generate the same data matrix and use the subroutine to create and print the three matrices.

```
                      m

   6.5321484 12.982739 7.8530913

                      s

   3.9110141 0.9280167 6.2611224

            standardized

    1.297565 -1.205853 1.7341685
   -0.332141 0.9480863 0.0595209
   -0.373861  0.369444  0.964047
    0.691142 -0.550814 -0.565355
    0.2616091 0.4027946 -1.076071
    0.0434776 -0.955056 1.0106784
   -1.930697 2.0156739 -1.022882
   -0.125782 0.3309627 0.4223396
   -0.919991 -0.532745  -1.05565
    1.3886794 -0.822494 -0.470797
```

4. **Using a SAS Data Set, Creating an IML Module, and Exporting Results to a New Data Table**

   a. Print the **govtDemand** data set and notice that each continuous variable has missing values.

   b. Read the **govtDemand** data set into an IML matrix named **govt**.

   c. Create a function that takes a vector as input and imputes all missing values with the mean of the vector and returns the imputed vector.

   d. Impute columns 2 through 4 and create a new SAS data set named **govtImputed**, with the same names as **govtDemand**, which contains the imputed matrix. Because a matrix is being exported to a SAS data set, be sure to use the COLNAME= option in the CREATE statement.

   e. Finally, print the SAS data set and also run PROC CORR on the variables **agric**, **manu**, and **labor**.

```
    submit;
        proc print data=sp4r.newGovt;run;
            proc corr data=sp4r.newGovt;
                var agric manu labor;
        run;
    endsubmit;
quit;
```

| Obs | YEAR | AGRIC | MANU | LABOR |
|-----|------|-------|------|-------|
| 1 | 1982 | 600.00 | 1000.00 | 600.00 |
| 2 | 1983 | 1100.00 | 1200.00 | 792.00 |
| 3 | 1984 | 1100.00 | 1350.00 | 800.00 |
| 4 | 1985 | 1150.00 | 1547.31 | 825.00 |
| 5 | 1986 | 1200.00 | 1475.00 | 850.00 |
| 6 | 1987 | 1272.92 | 1500.00 | 900.00 |
| 7 | 1988 | 1400.00 | 1650.00 | 920.00 |
| 8 | 1989 | 1420.00 | 1650.00 | 886.69 |
| 9 | 1990 | 1272.92 | 1680.00 | 940.00 |
| 10 | 1991 | 1450.00 | 1700.00 | 950.00 |
| 11 | 1992 | 1450.00 | 1720.00 | 975.00 |
| 12 | 1993 | 1460.00 | 1720.00 | 975.00 |
| 13 | 1994 | 1470.00 | 1730.00 | 1000.00 |
| 14 | 1995 | 1475.00 | 1740.00 | 1000.00 |

```
                          The CORR Procedure

             3  Variables:    AGRIC    MANU    LABOR

                          Simple Statistics

Variable      N         Mean      Std Dev        Sum       Minimum      Maximum

AGRIC        14         1273     239.90750      17821     600.00000        1475
MANU         14         1547     225.10353      21662          1000        1740
LABOR        14    886.69231     108.56999      12414     600.00000        1000


              Pearson Correlation Coefficients, N = 14
                     Prob > |r| under H0: Rho=0

                         AGRIC        MANU        LABOR

           AGRIC       1.00000     0.94119      0.96882
                                   <.0001       <.0001

           MANU        0.94119     1.00000      0.95092
                       <.0001                   <.0001

           LABOR       0.96882     0.95092      1.00000
                       <.0001      <.0001
```

5. **Calling Statistical Graphics from SAS/IML**

   a. Read the variables **saleprice**, **overall_qual**, **gr_liv_area**, **garage_area**, **basement_area**, **deck_porch_area**, and **age_sold** from the **AmesHousing** data set into an IML matrix named **imlAmes**.

   b. Create a correlation matrix from **imlAmes** named **corrAmes** and print it.

```
                           corrAmes

         1  0.7345057  0.6504636  0.5789207  0.6895635   0.439889  -0.615425
 0.7345057          1  0.5787329  0.3859067  0.4564424  0.2795069  -0.442376
 0.6504636  0.5787329          1  0.3328336  0.4398542  0.2805839  -0.192722
 0.5789207  0.3859067  0.3328336          1  0.3562982  0.2498748  -0.413458
 0.6895635  0.4564424  0.4398542  0.3562982          1  0.3368862   -0.39529
  0.439889  0.2795069  0.2805839  0.2498748  0.3368862          1  -0.205836
-0.615425  -0.442376  -0.192722  -0.413458   -0.39529  -0.205836          1
```

   c. Navigate to the SAS/IML documentation and review the HEATMAP subroutine. Create a heat map of the correlation matrix. Use the XVALUES= and YVALUES= options to set appropriate labels for the rows and columns of the plot. Also, provide the map with a title. Finally, change the color coding of the heat map to **"Temperature"**.

   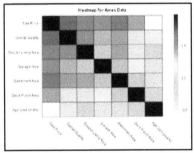

   d. Go to the **Work** directory and open the **_heatmap** data set. SAS/IML exported the data set required to be used by the SGPLOT procedure to create the heat map.

6. **Simulating the Birthday Problem**

   a. Use simulation to calculate the empirical probability of two people sharing the same birthdate in a group of 23 people. Use 1000 iterations. Assume that none of the people is born on Leap Day and every birthdate is equally likely.

   b. Invoke PROC IML, set the random seed, and begin a DO loop with 1000 simulations. Create a vector named **pair** to hold the results of each iteration.

   c. Draw 23 birthdates using the SAMPLE function. (Dates can be represented as the numbers 1 through 365.)

   d. Check whether any two birthdates are the same. (Hint: Use the UNIQUE function.)

   e. If at least two birthdates are the same, set the variable **pair** to 1. Otherwise, set **pair** to zero.

   f. Calculate the proportion of iterations in which a pair was found.

   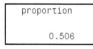

   ```
   proportion

         0.506
   ```

   g. How can you avoid using the DO loop for this simulation?

## Solutions

### Multiple Choice

1. a and c. There are two options for printing in SAS. First, you can assign a value to a matrix and then print the matrix. Second, if you do not want to create a new variable, you can use parentheses in the PRINT statement to print the specified value.

2. d. To find the mean of each row use the : operator in the second argument of the braces. To find the minimum of all elements of a matrix, you can use the >< symbol in each argument of the braces or simply use one >< symbol and ignore the comma.

3. b. A SAS/IML subroutine cannot be used in an assignment statement.

4. a, b, and d. To create a user-defined module, use the START and FINISH statement. Functions require the RETURN statement and can only return a single matrix. Subroutines on the other hand do not use the RETURN statement and can create multiple matrices. Also, functions require an assignment statement and subroutines cannot be used with an assignment statement. They are executed with either the CALL or RUN statements.

5. b. To specify the catalog that we want to create or call from, use the RESET STORAGE statement. To load a module and matrix back into your IML session use the LOAD statement and set the keyword MODULE equal to the desired modules in parentheses followed by your matrices.

6. a, b, and c. For answers A and B remember to use all three statements to do each task. Names of IML vectors are passed to the SAS data set as variable names. On the other hand, the user must set the names as an option in the CREATE statement to specify the data set variable names when passing a matrix to a data set. Otherwise, the SAS data set names default to COL1, COL2, COL3, and so on.

### Short Answer

1. In general, the LOC function returns a row vector containing indices of the elements in a matrix that satisfy a criterion. If an expression is not specified, the LOC function finds elements that are nonzero and nonmissing.

### Programming Exercises

1. **Practicing with Basic Operations**

   In this exercise, you perform operations on the data used in the previous demonstration. Use the code below at the beginning of the exercise program.

   ```
   proc iml;
   items =      {'Groceries','Utilities','Rent','Car Expenses',
                 'Fun Money','Personal Expenses'};
   weeks =      {'Week 1','Week 2','Week 3','Week 4'};
   amounts =    { 96   78   82   93,
                  61   77   62   68,
                 300  300  300  300,
                  25   27   98   18,
                  55   34   16   53,
                 110   85   96  118};
   weeklyIncome ={900 850 1050 950};
   weeklyExpenses=amounts[+,];
   ```

   a. Create a 1 x 4 matrix named **proportionIncomeSpent** whose elements are the proportion of each week's income that went to expenses. Use the RESET statement to suppress the automatic printing of matrix names. Print the **proportionIncomeSpent** matrix with the values of **weeks** used as column labels and PERCENT7.2 used as a format.

   ```
   proportionIncomeSpent=weeklyExpenses / weeklyIncome;
   reset noname;
   print "Proportion of income spent each week",
       proportionIncomeSpent[colname=weeks format=percent7.2];
   ```

PROC IML Output

```
 Proportion of income spent each week

   Week 1  Week 2  Week 3  Week 4

   71.9%   70.7%   62.3%   68.4%
```

b. Create a 1 x 4 matrix named **proportionIncomeSaved** whose elements are equal to the proportion of each week's income that did not go to expenses. That is, use an implicit loop to subtract the values of **proportionIncomeSpent** from one. Print the **proportionIncomeSaved** matrix with the values of weeks used as column labels and PERCENT7.2 used as a format.

```
proportionIncomeSaved=1 - proportionIncomeSpent;
print "Proportion of income saved each week",
    proportionIncomeSaved[colname=weeks format=percent7.2];
```

PROC IML Output

```
Proportion of income saved each week

   Week 1  Week 2  Week 3  Week 4

   28.1%   29.3%   37.7%   31.6%
```

c. Create a 6 x 4 matrix named **proportionSpentPerItem** whose elements are the proportion of each week's income spent on each item, by week. That is, use an implicit loop to divide the **amounts** matrix by the **weeklyIncome** matrix. Print the **proportionSpentPerItem** matrix with the values of **items** used as row labels, the values of **weeks** used as column labels, and PERCENT7.2 used as a format.

```
proportionSpentPerItem=amounts/weeklyIncome;
print "Percentage of income spent on each item, by week",
    proportionSpentPerItem [rowname=items
    colname=weeks format=percent7.2];
```

```
 Percentage of income spent on each item, by week
                    Week 1  Week 2  Week 3  Week 4

Groceries           10.7%   9.18%   7.81%   9.79%
Utilities           6.78%   9.06%   5.90%   7.16%
Rent                33.3%   35.3%   28.6%   31.6%
Car Expenses        2.78%   3.18%   9.33%   1.89%
Fun Money           6.11%   4.00%   1.52%   5.58%
Personal Expenses   12.2%   10.0%   9.14%   12.4%
```

d. Create a matrix named **weeklyExpenseChange** with the same number of rows as **amounts** but with one less column than **amounts** (in other words, a 6 x 3 matrix). Fill it with missing numeric values. This should be done with a matrix literal. Fill each column of **weeklyExpenseChange** with each column of **amounts** minus the previous column of **amounts**. That is, column 1 of **weeklyExpenseChange** should equal column 2 of **amounts** minus column 1 of **amounts**, and so on. Print a title and print the matrix. Use columns 2 through 4 of **weeks** as column labels and use **items** as row labels.

```
weeklyExpenseChange={. . .,
                     . . .,
                     . . .,
                     . . .,
                     . . .,
                     . . .};
weeklyExpenseChange [,1]=amounts[,2] - amounts[,1];
weeklyExpenseChange [,2]=amounts[,3] - amounts[,2];
weeklyExpenseChange [,3]=amounts[,4] - amounts[,3];
print "Change in spending from previous week, by item",
    weeklyExpenseChange [rowname=items
    colname={"Week 2","Week 3", "Week 4"}];
quit;
```

```
Change in spending from previous week, by item
                     Week 2     Week 3     Week 4

Groceries              -18          4         11
Utilities               16        -15          6
Rent                     0          0          0
Car Expenses             2         71        -80
Fun Money              -21        -18         37
Personal Expenses      -25         11         22
```

2. **Generating a Multiple Regression Data Matrix and Computing Parameter Estimates**

   This exercise extends the ideas from the previous demonstration.

   a. Generate data from a multiple regression model, $y_i = \beta_0 + \beta_1 x_{1i} + \beta_2 x_{2i} + \varepsilon_i$ , with 20 samples where $\beta_0 = 3$ , $\beta_1 = 2$ , $\beta_2 = -1$, and $\varepsilon_i \sim N(0, \sigma = 5)$ . Let $x_{1i} \sim Uniform(0,20)$ and $x_{2i} \sim Uniform(10,30)$ . Use the seed 27606 to duplicate your results. Generate the random numbers using the RANDFUN function. Print the generated values.

```
proc iml;
    call randseed(27606);
    n = 20;
    beta0 = 3;
    beta1 = 2;
    beta2 = -1;
    xvals1 = randfun(n,"Uniform");
    xvals1 = xvals1*20;
    xvals2 = randfun(n,"Uniform");
    xvals2 = (xvals2*20) + 10;
    error = randfun(n,"Normal",0,5);
    y = beta0 + beta1*xvals1 + beta2*xvals2 + error;
    print y beta0 beta1 beta2 xvals1 xvals2 error;
```

| y | beta0 | beta1 | beta2 | xvals1 | xvals2 | error |
|---|---|---|---|---|---|---|
| 2.3890519 | 3 | 2 | 1 | 15.535752 | 25.086444 | 6.596008 |
| 27.055062 | | | | 19.109842 | 16.338432 | 2.1718106 |
| -4.292507 | | | | 8.7436082 | 21.76381 | -3.015913 |
| 11.835473 | | | | 12.034105 | 20.732266 | 5.4995483 |
| 18.823426 | | | | 12.89481 | 16.240074 | 6.2738806 |
| -26.1453 | | | | 1.948081 | 23.511204 | -9.530258 |
| 27.55394 | | | | 10.206666 | 15.207025 | 1.3476321 |
| 15.761662 | | | | 14.474217 | 17.647193 | 1.460422 |
| 12.815418 | | | | 12.986986 | 18.152577 | 1.9940234 |
| 19.421855 | | | | 18.214594 | 25.124106 | 5.1167724 |
| 16.696806 | | | | 15.184676 | 29.289954 | 12.617408 |
| 15.49262 | | | | 2.9719555 | 27.424333 | 2.9878057 |
| 6.7790585 | | | | 15.249747 | 20.255946 | -6.464469 |
| 31.024149 | | | | 19.654065 | 11.005698 | 0.276282 |
| 6.8295732 | | | | 9.9692864 | 27.152395 | 11.043396 |
| -8.10431 | | | | 0.0501745 | 11.999825 | 0.795106 |
| -10.70045 | | | | 1.934529 | 16.587159 | -0.982352 |
| 28.096877 | | | | 19.974169 | 10.011983 | -4.839478 |
| 5.1143731 | | | | 9.217378 | 13.189886 | 3.130499 |
| 6.3452045 | | | | 16.397849 | 27.952028 | -1.498465 |

   b. Create the design matrix and compute $\hat{\beta} = (X^T X)^- X^T Y$ using the INV function. Print your results.

```
x = j(n,1,1)||xvals1||xvals2;
betaHat = inv(x`*x)*(x`*y);
print x, betaHat;
*Alternative SAS Function;
*betaHat = solve( (x`*x)*(x`*y) );
*print betaHat;
```

```
             X

1 6.9833149 28.419994
1 11.619663  13.11864
1 14.863959 25.720417
1 17.563605 14.31566
1 0.0771578 24.440131
1   16.60792 26.879481
1 14.251058 18.034902
1 14.773279 12.525219
1 1.6650986 29.064125
1 11.628301 10.744335
1  14.12347 19.860202
1 1.5470275 20.552019
1    19.547 25.236564
1 12.918223 29.589143
1 1.3057281  18.96901
1  8.558932 16.789311
1 6.7389815 20.715758
1  0.425611 20.222944
1 0.1731237 10.720545
1 13.190648 22.985184


   betaHat

   4.5097506
   2.0297133
   -1.040226
```

c.  Compute and print the estimates $\widehat{\sigma}^2$ and $\widehat{\sigma}$ where $\widehat{\sigma}^2 = \dfrac{\sum\limits_{i=1}^{n}\left(y_i - \widehat{y_i}\right)}{n-1}$ . Recall that SAS does

not use the ^ operator to exponentiate matrix elements.

```
      pred = x*betaHat;
      sse = sum( (y-pred)##2 );
      sigma2Hat = sse / (n-1);
      sigmaHat = sqrt(sigma2Hat);
      print sigma2Hat sigmaHat;
quit;
```

```
sigma2Hat  sigmaHat

33.790635 5.8129713
```

3.  **Creating User-Defined Functions and Subroutines**

Standardized values are computed as $\dfrac{x - \overline{x}}{std(x)}$ where $std(x) = \sqrt{\dfrac{\sum\left(x - \overline{x}\right)}{n-1}}$ .

a.  Create a function, STANDARDIZE, that takes a matrix as an input and returns the matrix with each column standardized.

```
proc iml;
    start standardize(x);
        n=nrow(x);
        mean=x[:,];              /* means for all columns */
        xbar=repeat(mean,n,1); /* n rows of means */
        x=x-xbar;                /* center x to mean zero */
        stdv=std(x);     /* standard deviations for columns */
        x=x/stdv;              /* scale to std dev 1 */
        return(x);
    finish;
```

The mean of each column here is computed using the reduction operator [ :, ].

b.  Create a 10 x 3 matrix of random numbers where the first column is 123, the second column is 123, and the third column is 123. Use the seed 802 to duplicate your results. Print the matrix and then use the STANDARDIZE function to create and print the standardized matrix.

```
      n = 10;
      call randseed(802);
      mymat = randfun(n,"Normal",5,5)
          ||randfun(n,"Uniform",10,15)
          ||randfun(n,"Exponential",7);
```

```
        print mymat;
        stand = standardize(mymat);
        print stand;
quit;
```

```
                mymat

11.606944 11.863687 18.710933
5.2331384 13.862579 8.2257589
5.0699716 13.325589 13.889108
9.2352147 12.471574 4.3133361
7.5553052 13.356539 1.1156816
6.7021899 12.096431 14.181072
-1.018837 14.853318 1.4487006
6.0402131 13.289878 10.497412
2.9340508 12.488342 1.2435366
11.963293 12.219451 4.9053748

                stand

1.297565 -1.205853 1.7341685
-0.332141 0.9480863 0.0595209
-0.373861 0.369444 0.964047
0.691142 -0.550814 -0.565355
0.2616091 0.4027946 -1.076071
0.0434776 -0.955056 1.0106784
-1.930697 2.0156739 -1.022882
-0.125782 0.3309627 0.4223396
-0.919991 -0.532745 -1.05565
1.3886794 -0.822494 -0.470797
```

c.  Alter the STANDARDIZE function and create the subroutine STANDSUB. Let the subroutine take a matrix as input and output the standardized matrix, as well as the column means and standard deviations.

```
proc iml;
    start standsub(stand,mean,stdv,x);
        n=nrow(x);
        mean=x[:,];                /* means for all columns */
        xbar=repeat(mean,n,1); /* n rows of means */
        x=x-xbar;                  /* center x to mean zero */
        stdv=std(x);     /* standard deviations for columns */
        stand=x/stdv;            /* scale to std dev 1 */
    finish;
```

d.  Generate the same data matrix and use the subroutine to create and print the three matrices.

```
    n = 10;
    call randseed(802);
    mymat = randfun(n,"Normal",5,5)
        ||randfun(n,"Uniform",10,15)
        ||randfun(n,"Exponential",7);
    call standsub(standardized,m,s,mymat);
    print m, s, standardized;
quit;
```

```
                m

6.5321484 12.982739 7.8530913

                s

3.9110141 0.9280167 6.2611224

            standardized

1.297565 -1.205853 1.7341685
-0.332141 0.9480863 0.0595209
-0.373861 0.369444 0.964047
0.691142 -0.550814 -0.565355
0.2616091 0.4027946 -1.076071
0.0434776 -0.955056 1.0106784
-1.930697 2.0156739 -1.022882
-0.125782 0.3309627 0.4223396
-0.919991 -0.532745 -1.05565
1.3886794 -0.822494 -0.470797
```

4. **Using a SAS Data Set, Creating an IML Module, and Exporting Results to a New Data Table**

    a.  Print the **govtDemand** data set and notice that each continuous variable has missing values.

    ```
    proc print data=sp4r.govtDemand;
    run;
    ```

    | Obs | year | agric | manu | labor |
    |-----|------|-------|------|-------|
    | 1 | 1982 | 600 | 1000 | 600 |
    | 2 | 1983 | 1100 | 1200 | 792 |
    | 3 | 1984 | 1100 | 1350 | 800 |
    | 4 | 1985 | 1150 | . | 825 |
    | 5 | 1986 | 1200 | 1475 | 850 |
    | 6 | 1987 | . | 1500 | 900 |
    | 7 | 1988 | 1400 | 1650 | 920 |
    | 8 | 1989 | 1420 | 1650 | . |
    | 9 | 1990 | . | 1680 | 940 |
    | 10 | 1991 | 1450 | 1700 | 950 |
    | 11 | 1992 | 1450 | 1720 | 975 |
    | 12 | 1993 | 1460 | 1720 | 975 |
    | 13 | 1994 | 1470 | 1730 | 1000 |
    | 14 | 1995 | 1475 | 1740 | 1000 |

    b.  Read the **govtDemand** data set into an IML matrix named **govt**.

    ```
    proc iml;
        use sp4r.govtDemand;
        read all into govt;
        close sp4r.govtDemand;
    ```

    c.  Create a function that takes a vector as input and imputes all missing values with the mean of the vector and returns the imputed vector.

    ```
    start impute(colvec);
        colvec[loc(colvec=.)] = mean(colvec);
        return(colvec);
    finish impute;
    ```

    The LOC function is to find the index of all missing values in the vector.

    d.  Impute columns 2 through 4 and create a new SAS data set named **govtImputed**, with the same names as **govtDemand**, which contains the imputed matrix. Because a matrix is being exported to a SAS data set, be sure to use the COLNAME= option in the CREATE statement.

    ```
    govtImputed = govt[,1]||impute(govt[,2])
        ||impute(govt[,3])||impute(govt[,4]);
    create sp4r.newGovt from govtImputed
        [colname={year, agric, manu, labor}];
    append from govtImputed;
    close sp4r.newGovt;
    ```

    e.  Finally, print the SAS data set and also run PROC CORR on the variables **agric, manu,** and **labor**.

    ```
        submit;
            proc print data=sp4r.newGovt;run;
                proc corr data=sp4r.newGovt;
                    var agric manu labor;
            run;
        endsubmit;
    quit;
    ```

```
                        The CORR Procedure

              3  Variables:    AGRIC    MANU    LABOR

                        Simple Statistics

Variable      N       Mean      Std Dev        Sum     Minimum     Maximum

AGRIC        14       1273     239.90750      17821   600.00000      1475
MANU         14       1547     225.10353      21662      1000        1740
LABOR        14   886.69231    108.56999      12414   600.00000      1000

              Pearson Correlation Coefficients, N = 14
                    Prob > |r| under H0: Rho=0

                       AGRIC        MANU        LABOR

          AGRIC      1.00000     0.94119      0.96682
                                  <.0001       <.0001

          MANU       0.94119     1.00000      0.95092
                      <.0001                   <.0001

          LABOR      0.96682     0.95092      1.00000
                      <.0001      <.0001
```

5. **Calling Statistical Graphics from SAS/IML**

   a.  Read the variables **saleprice**, **overall_qual**, **gr_liv_area**, **garage_area**, **basement_area**, **deck_porch_area**, and **age_sold** from the **AmesHousing** data set into an IML matrix named **imlAmes**.

```
proc iml;
    use sp4r.ameshousing;
    read all var {saleprice overall_qual gr_liv_area
        garage_area basement_area deck_porch_area age_sold}
        into imlAmes;
    close sp4r.ameshousing;
```

   b.  Create a correlation matrix from **imlAmes** named **corrAmes** and print it.

```
corrAmes = corr(imlAmes);
print corrAmes;
```

```
                              corrAmes

        1 0.7345057 0.6504636 0.5789207 0.6895635  0.439889 -0.615425
0.7345057         1 0.5787329 0.3859067 0.4564424 0.2795069 -0.442376
0.6504636 0.5787329         1 0.3328336 0.4398542 0.2805839 -0.192722
0.5789207 0.3859067 0.3328336         1 0.3562982 0.2498748 -0.413458
0.6895635 0.4564424 0.4398542 0.3562982         1 0.3368862  -0.39529
 0.439889 0.2795069 0.2805839 0.2498748 0.3368862         1 -0.205836
-0.615425 -0.442376 -0.192722 -0.413458  -0.39529 -0.205836         1
```

   c.  Navigate to the SAS/IML documentation and review the HEATMAP subroutine. Create a heat map of the correlation matrix. Use the XVALUES= and YVALUES= options to set appropriate labels for the rows and columns of the plot. Also, provide the map with a title. Finally, change the color coding of the heat map to **"Temperature"**.

```
    varNames = {"Sale Price" "Overall Quality"
        "Ground Living Area" "Garage Area" "Basement Area"
        "Deck Porch Area" "Age Sold (years)" };
    call heatmapcont(corrAmes) xvalues=varNames
        yvalues=varNames
      colorramp="Temperature" title="Heatmap for Ames Data";
quit;
```

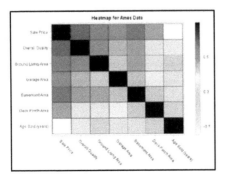

d. Go to the **Work** directory and open the **_heatmap** data set. SAS/IML exported the data set required to be used by the SGPLOT procedure to create the heat map.

6. **Simulating the Birthday Problem**

Use simulation to calculate the empirical probability of two people sharing the same birthdate in a group of 23 people. Use 1000 iterations. Assume that none of the people is born on Leap Day and every birthdate is equally likely.

a. Invoke PROC IML, set the random seed, and begin a DO loop with 1000 simulations. Create a vector named **pair** to hold the results of each iteration.

```
proc iml;
    n=23;
    numberIterations=1000;
    call randseed(802);
    pair = j(numberIterations,1,.);
    do iteration=1 to numberIterations;
```

b. Draw 23 birthdates using the SAMPLE function. (Dates can be represented as the numbers 1 through 365.)

```
dates = 1:365;
birthDates=sample(dates,n);
```

c. Check whether any two birthdates are the same. (Hint: Use the UNIQUE function.)

```
uniqueDates=unique(birthDates);
```

d. If at least two birthdates are the same, set the variable **pair** to 1. Otherwise, set **pair** to zero.

```
    if ncol(uniqueDates) < n then pair[iteration]=1;
    else pair[iteration]=0;
end;
```

e. Calculate the proportion of iterations in which a pair was found.

```
    proportion=pair[:];
    print proportion;
quit;
```

```
proportion

  0.506
```

f. How can you avoid using the DO loop for this simulation?

Simulate dates in a matrix with dimension (number of iterations) by (number of people).

```
proc iml;
    n=23;
    numberIterations=1000;
    call randseed(23571113);
    prob=j(364,1,1/365);
    birthDates=j(numberIterations,n,.);
    call randgen(birthDates,"Table",prob);
```

After you enter IML and set the random number seed, this version of the birthday problem simulation creates a vector of probabilities, **prob**, to be used as a parameter for the table distribution. The program then creates a 1000 x 23 matrix of missing values and assigns it to **birthDates**. The program then fills the **birthDates** matrix with values drawn from the table distribution with parameter **prob**.

```
    rowUnique=countunique(birthDates,"ROW");
    proportion=(rowUnique < n)[+] / numberIterations;
    print proportion;
quit;
```

Specifying the "ROW" option for **countunique** tells the function to calculate the number of unique elements in each row of the argument matrix. Then **rowUnique** is assigned the number of unique birthdates for each row in **birthDates**. The syntax **(rowUnique < n) [+]** counts the number of rows that contain fewer than 23 unique birthdates. Dividing the number of unique birthdates by the number of iterations provides the proportion of samples containing at least two matching birthdates.

# Chapter 8: A Bridge Between SAS and R

## Introduction

SAS views open-source software as a complementary resource, and SAS has been using open-source software for years. For example, it has used Perl, SQL, and others. R is just the newest open-source software, which happens to be able to create models as well, but you can assimilate open-source tools into your SAS script to enjoy the benefits.

Working with R from SAS is incredibly easy. SAS provides a seamless interface between the two languages. You can write R code directly in the SAS code editor as if you were in R studio, send the code to R, run an analysis in R, and return the results. You can do all this with a click of a button. Because you know R and now you are comfortable working with the interactive matrix language, in this chapter you will learn about the four subroutines that you need to use to move your code and data back and forth between SAS and R. In this chapter, you will see that you can freely write R code within a SAS script, send it to the open-source software R, and retrieve the results.

If there is a new package you really want to try in R, SAS gives you a very seamless interface to do that directly in SAS. You can compare methods, because of course, all algorithms are data dependent. And you can create a diverse set of plots. You can integrate open-source software into three different SAS environments.

The easiest way to work with R is in the interactive matrix language. You can write open-source code directly in the SUBMITBLOCK that we saw in Chapter 7; we just have to give it the R option. A second method is to execute open-source code via a DATA Step in Base SAS. This can be challenging. It requires using Java as an intermediary tool, which means you pass your code to Java, and then Java is going to pass that code to R. Another alternative is to use system commands. Finally, if you are familiar with Enterprise Miner, you can execute open-source code via the Open Source Integration node.

# Calling SAS from IML

## Readying Your Machine to Call R

In order to work with R inside SAS, we need to enable R language statements. To see whether RLANG is enabled on your machine, you can run Program 8.1 and ask the OPTIONS procedure if the option= to RLANG is on.

**Program 8.1: RLANG**

```
proc options option=rlang;
run;
```

One of two results will be printed to the log. You will either get a NORLANG, meaning you do not have permission to call R from SAS, or you will get RLANG, meaning you do have permission to call R from SAS.

How do you turn a NORLANG into an RLANG? The easiest way is just to right-click the SAS icon on your desktop. Notice in the Target field, as shown in Figure 8.1, it provides the location of your SAS configuration file. Generally, it is at this location: C:\ProgramFiles\SASHome\ SASFoundation\9.4\nls\en\sasv9.cfg".

**Figure 8.1: SAS Properties**

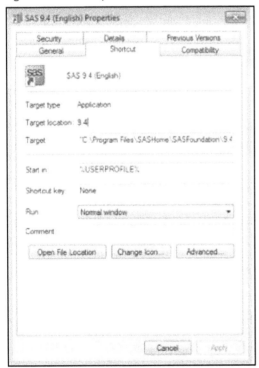

Navigate to the SASV9.CFG file and open it. When you are in the configuration file, add -RLANG at the bottom as shown in Figure 8.2. Save these changes. Make sure that SAS is not open because SAS calls the configuration file each time it starts.

Figure 8.2: Configuration File

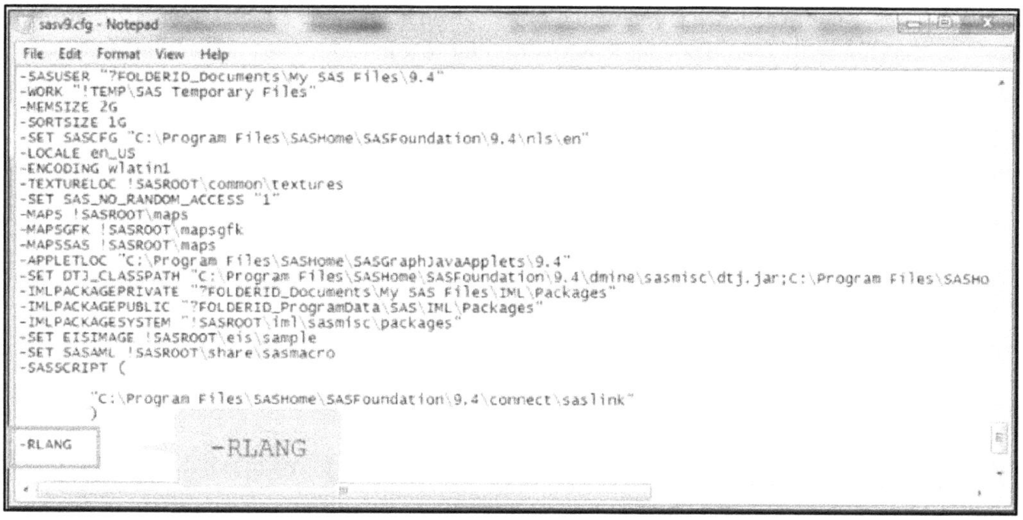

Once you have altered your configuration file and enabled R language statements, you can do the following:

- send IML matrices in SAS data sets to R

- submit R code in the IML script

- return R results from analyses as IML matrices or SAS data sets

> **Tip:** To run R with SAS, R must be installed on the same machine as SAS. Because SAS University Edition installs on a virtual machine where R cannot be installed, R cannot be used with SAS University Edition.

## Subroutines

To work with R in SAS, there are four subroutines that you need to be familiar with:

- EXPORTDATASETTOR

- EXPORTMATRIXTOR

- IMPORTMATRIXFROMR

- MPORTDATASETFROMR

Let's look at each of these in more detail.

### Exporting SAS Data Sets

The first subroutine is EXPORTDATASETTOR, and it does exactly what you would expect from its name. It exports your SAS data set to R as an R data frame using the following syntax:

**CALL EXPORTDATASETTOR**("*SAS-data-set*", "*R-data-frame*");

The first argument is the SAS data set. The second is the R data frame that you are going to refer to in code. The helpful thing about this subroutine is, it exports the SAS data set variables to the R data frame as column names.

## Exporting IML Matrices

Again, EXPORTMATRIXTOR, does exactly what you would expect given its name. It exports your IML matrix to an R matrix, and you can choose the name of your R matrix to refer to it in code. As shown in the following syntax:

**CALL EXPORTMATRIXTOR**(*IML-matrix*, "*R-matrix*");

## Submitting R Syntax

To submit code to R, you are going to use a Submit block, and after the forward slash in the Submit statement, you are going to use the R option as shown in the following syntax:

**SUBMIT / R;**
 *R statements*
**ENDSUBMIT;**

Using this syntax tells SAS to submit this code directly to R. Otherwise, it tries to run it as if it were SAS code.

Program 8.2 gives an example of exporting a matrix and submitting code to R.

**Program 8.2: Submit R Code**
```
imlMatrix = {0 1, 1 2, 3 5, 8 13};
call ExportMatrixToR(imlMatrix,"rmatrix");
submit / R;
    print(rmatrix)
endsubmit;
```

In Program 8.2, we are creating a four by two matrix, exporting that matrix to R, and giving it the name rmatrix. We are submitting only one line of code, just print rmatrix in the R console.

All R command line output is automatically returned to SAS and displayed in the results viewer. The format that it prints it in is exactly the same as R. So Output 8.2 shows that the matrix printed in R, and it prints the same thing in the results viewer of SAS.

**Output 8.2: Results of Program 8.2**
```
   A1 A2
[1,] 0  1
[2,] 1  2
[3,] 3  5
[4,] 8 13
```

## Importing R Objects into IML Matrices

To get results in R back into SAS to view them, we can use the IMPORTMATRIXFROMR subroutine to import an R object to a new IML matrix name of your choosing with the following syntax:

**CALL IMPORTMATRIXFROMR**(*IML-matrix*, "*R-object*");

Program 8.3 is an example of exporting from SAS to R and back again.

**Program 8.3: SAS to R and Back**
```
imlMatrix = {0 1, 1 2, 3 5, 8 13};
call ExportMatrixToR(imlMatrix,"rmatrix");
submit / R;
    rmatrix = rmatrix + 49
endsubmit;
call ImportMatrixFromR(NewMatrix,"rmatrix");
print NewMatrix;
```

In Program 8.3 we have the same four by two matrix that we used in Program 8.2. We export that matrix to R with the name rmatrix and submit one line of code to add 49 to every element of that R matrix. Then, we import that matrix from R with the appropriate subroutine with the new IML matrix name, NewMatrix. Now we have access to use it in SAS and can print it in SAS format as shown in Output 8.3.

**Output 8.3: Results of Program 8.3**

| NewMatrix | |
|---|---|
| 49 | 50 |
| 50 | 51 |
| 52 | 54 |
| 57 | 62 |

### Importing R Objects into SAS Data Sets

Finally, you can return your R data frame as a SAS data set with the IMPORTDATASETFROMR subroutine using the following syntax:

**CALL IMPORTDATASETFROMR**("*SAS-data-set*", "*R-object*");

You can name your SAS data set whatever you would like. When you work with data sets in this environment, the R data frame column names are returned as SAS data set variable names so that you don't have to rename anything.

# Calling R from Base SAS Java API

As mentioned in the introduction to this chapter, you can write and submit R code inside a DATA step. However, the SAS DATA step does not pass an R script directly from SAS to R. JAVA must be used as an intermediate tool. This path is not inherent. You must manually create the connection from SAS to Java to R.

## Setup

First, Download and extract the project ZIP file SAS_Base_OpenSrcIntegration.zip from https://communities.sas.com/docs/DOC-10746. The download prompts you to save the files on your computer at C:\SGF2015\OpenSrcIntegration. The subsequent steps assume that this is the location of the Java files.

## Connect SAS to R

Next, download the Java Development Kit (JDK) from oracle.com. Downloading the Java Development Kit gives you access to the JAVAC command on the Windows command line. The JAVAC command is used to compile the extracted Java files, and creates the connection from SAS to R.

Once you have downloaded the JDK, follow these steps to compile the Java classes and complete setup:

1. Open the Windows command line.
2. Enter the following
   a. cd C:\SGF2015\OpenSrcIntegration
   b. – "C:\Program Files\Java\jdk1.7.0_25\bin\javac"
      src/dev/* -d bin

3. Add the following location of the compiled Java classes to the SAS configuration file. C:\Program Files\SASHome\SASFoundation\9.4\nls\en\sasv9.cfg. (This is the same SAS configuration file that is used to add the RLANG option from the previous section.)

    a. -SET CLASSPATH "C:\SGF2015\OpenSrcIntegration\bin"

4. Ensure that the Java classes are compiled and that the CLASSPATH is set correctly.

    a. Set a working directory and the Java directory.

```
%let WORK_DIR = C:\SGF2015\OpenSrcIntegration;
%let JAVA_BIN_DIR = &WORK_DIR.\bin;
```

    b. Validate the Java pipeline.

```
data _null_;
    length _x1 $ 32767;
    _x1 = sysget('CLASSPATH');
    _x2 = index(upcase(trim(_x1)),
        %upcase("&JAVA_BIN_DIR"));
    if _x2 = 0 then put "ERROR: Invalid Java
        Classpath.";
run;
```

If the Java pipeline is created correctly, the SAS log is empty. Otherwise, the log contains "ERROR: Invalid Java Classpath." Now you are ready to submit R code inside a DATA step!

## R Command Line

The next step sets the R system location. Right-click the R desktop icon on your computer and select Properties. Copy the value from the Target field shown in Figure 8.3.

**Figure 8.3: R Properties**

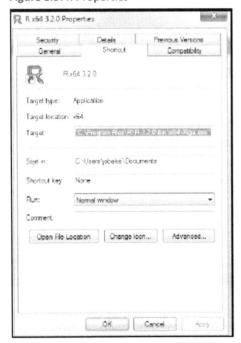

Paste the value from the Target field into SAS and create a macro variable. Replace the Rgui text with Rscript, as shown below:

```
%let R_EXEC_COMMAND =C:\Program Files\R\R-3.2.0\bin\x64\Rscript.exe;
```

Changing the text to Rscript sets the path to the R command line. This location tells Java where to pass the DATA step R script.

### DATA Step Syntax

The DATA step in Program 8.4 is used to submit R code. Add your R script to the R SCRIPT field.

**Program 8.4: DATA Step to Submit R Code**

```
data _NULL_;
    length rtn_val 8;
    length r_call $ 32000;

    r_expr = "-e";
    r_script = "R SCRIPT";

    r_call = catt('"', r_expr, '" "', r_script, '"');

    declare javaobjj("dev.SASJavaExec", "&R_EXEC_COMMAND",r_call);

    j.callIntMethod("executeProcess", rtn_val);
run;
```

> **Tip:** R command line output is returned to the SAS log in SAS format.

The DATA step method of calling R is unable to do either of the following tasks:

- Send a SAS data set to R.
- Return a matrix or data frame to a SAS data set.

If you want to send a SAS data set to R, you can use the EXPORT procedure to save data outside of the SAS environment. Read in the data file using an R statement. If you want to return a matrix or data frame to a SAS data set, you can save the matrix or data frame in R and use a PROC IMPORT statement to create a SAS data set.

### Writing R Script

When writing R script, you must end each R statement with a semicolon and use single quotation marks only. Remember that in R, double quotation marks are used to begin and end R script.

Program 8.5 shows an example of writing R script in a DATA step.

**Program 8.5: Partial DATA Step Code**

```
data _NULL_;
    ...
    r_script = "library(fields);
    setwd('C:/SGF2015/OpenSrcIntegration');
    locations = read.csv('locations.csv');
    dist_mat = rdist(locations);
    write.table(dist_mat,'dist_mat.csv',
        sep = ',',row.names=F);";
    ...
run;
```

The R script is condensed by removing all trailing blanks and is then concatenated with the –e variable. (This is done using the CATT function.) Thus, the R script sent to Java is as follows:

```
"-e library(fields);setwd('C:/SGF2015/OpenSrcIntegration');…"
```

The only blank is between the **–e** and the rest of the script. This is why it is necessary to use a semicolon after each statement. The R script is passed to R on a single line.

Program 8.5 begins by unpacking the fields R package. The read.csv() function reads in the locations data set in the directory specified in the setwd() function. PROC EXPORT can be used to export a SAS data set to a CSV and the directory can be chosen. The rdist() function creates a results matrix of the Euclidean distances between each location pair. Finally, the write.table() function exports the R results back to the working directory set by the setwd() function. Thus, the DATA step runs properly if the results from R are stored in the desired directory. The results can then be returned to SAS using PROC IMPORT.

## Calling R Script

Alternatively, you can use a DATA step to call and run a saved R script. Program 8.6 runs the dist.R file. Add the DECLARE JAVAOBJ and J.CALLINTMETHOD statements to the end of the DATA step.

**Program 8.6: Partial DATA Step Code**

```
data _null_;
    length rtn_val 8;
     r_pgm = "&WORK_DIR.\dist.R";
     r_arg1 = "&WORK_DIR";
     r_call = cat('"', trim(r_pgm), '" "',trim(r_arg1), '"');
     ...
run;
```

The rdist.R file is simply a saved R file. It does not require quoting the R code or using semicolons. The code from Program 8.6 would be saved as follows:

> **library(fields)**
> **setwd('C:/SGF2015/OpenSrcIntegration')**
> **locations = read.csv('locations.csv')**
> **dist_mat = rdist(locations)**
> **write.table(dist_mat,'dist_mat.csv',sep = ',',row.names=F)**

# Calling R from SAS Enterprise Miner

The SAS Enterprise Miner interface streamlines and simplifies common tasks associated with applied analysis. You can freely write R code within SAS Enterprise Miner's Open Source Integration node, send it to R, and retrieve the results.

The process flow in Figure 8.4 indicates each step in the analysis from data entry to modeling the data.

**Figure 8.4: Enterprise Miner Process Flow**

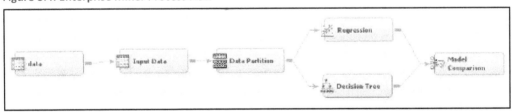

SAS Enterprise Miner has a point-and-click interface. It offers secure analysis management and provides a wide variety of tools with a consistent graphical interface. You can customize it by incorporating your choice of analysis methods and tools. The SAS Enterprise Miner tools that are available to your analysis are contained in the tools palette. The tools palette is arranged according to a process for data mining, SEMMA. SEMMA is an acronym for the following words:

- **S**ample—You sample the data by creating one or more data tables. The samples should be large enough to contain the significant information, but small enough to process.

- **E**xplore—You explore the data by searching for anticipated relationships, unanticipated trends, and anomalies in order to gain understanding and ideas.

- **M**odify—You modify the data by creating, selecting, and transforming the variables to focus the model selection process.

- **M**odel—You model the data by using the analytical tools to search for a combination of the data that reliably predicts a desired outcome.

- **A**ssess—You assess competing predictive models. (You build charts to evaluate the usefulness and reliability of the findings from the data mining process.)

Figure 8.5 shows the Tools Palette in SAS Enterprise Miner. It has tabs that correspond to each step of the SEMMA process as well as other tabs, including the Utility tab, that are helpful.

**Figure 8.5: Tools Palette**

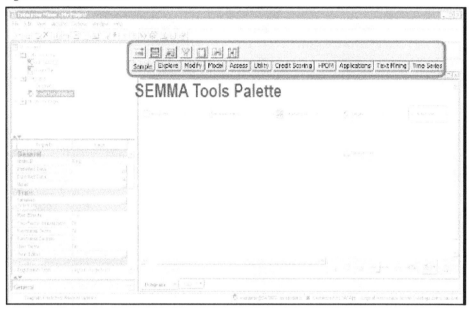

Additional tools are available in the Utility group. There are also specialized group tools, namely, HPDM (High-Performance Data Mining), Applications, and Time Series. With additional licensing, Credit Scoring and Text Mining groups are also available. All tool groups are discussed on the next several pages.

## Model Tab

The Model tab is a good starting location for new SAS Enterprise Miner users. The Regression tool enables you to fit both linear and logistic regression models to your data. You can use continuous, ordinal, and binary target variables. You can use both continuous and discrete variables as inputs. The tool supports the stepwise, forward, and backward selection methods. The interface enables you to create higher-order modeling terms such as polynomial terms and interactions.

## Utility Tab

The Open Source Integration tool can be found under the Utility Tab. It enables you to write code in the R language inside SAS Enterprise Miner by adding an Open Source Integration node to your process flow. The tool makes SAS Enterprise Miner data and metadata available to your R code and returns R results to SAS Enterprise Miner. In addition to training and scoring supervised and unsupervised R models, the Open Source Integration node enables data transformation and data exploration.

The SAS Code tool enables you to incorporate new or existing SAS code into process flow diagrams. The ability to write SAS code enables you to include additional SAS procedures into your data mining analysis. You can also use a SAS DATA step to create customized scoring code, to conditionally process data, and to concatenate or merge existing data sets. The tool provides a macro facility to dynamically reference data sets that are used for training, validation, testing, or scoring variables, such as input, target, and predict variables. After you run the SAS Code tool, the results and the data sets can then be exported for use by subsequent tools in the diagram.

## Open Source Integration Node

The Open Source Integration node enables the writing and use of R code in Enterprise Miner. It transfers data and results automatically between Enterprise Miner and R. All R packages must be installed in R before using the Open Source Integration node.

The Open Source Integration node requires you to

- enable R language statements in the SASV9.cfg file
- match the appropriate versions of SAS, R, and the PMML R package.

The Open Source Integration node is verified to work with 64-bit R. (32-bit R is not recommended.) The SYSCC=10 error indicates that the appropriate versions of SAS, R, and PMML are not being used. The user should uninstall the PMML package (or R, or both) and download the appropriate version.

## Output Mode

The Output mode specifies different ways that the output from the R code is available. Options are PMML, Merge, or None. Output mode None is used primarily to debug the R code and ensure that it is working properly. The log provides more detail about errors when output mode None is specified.

### PMML

Predictive Modeling Markup Language (PMML) is an open standard that enables certain R models to be translated into SAS DATA step code.

Here are the currently supported R models:

- linear models (lm)
- multinomial log-linear models (multinom)
- generalized linear models (glm)
- decision trees (rpart)
- neural networks (nnet)
- K-means clustering (kmeans)

### Merge

Merging the output mode enables integration with the thousands of R packages that are not supported in the PMML output mode. Variables created in R are merged with the SAS Enterprise Miner data source by the user. SAS DATA step code is not created.

The Merge mode is commonly used when applying the predict() function to the R model object. The predict() function returns results and merges the results to the workflow data set.

## Variable Handles

Enterprise Miner variable handles are used to efficiently create an R script. The words NUM and CLASS in a variable handle refer to numeric or categorical variables. A single INPUT variable handle refers to the entire set of numeric or categorical variables to be used as inputs.

Here are the variable handles:

- &EMR_MODEL—refers to the R model object.
- &EMR_NUM_TARGET and &EMR_CLASS_TARGET—refer to the response variable.

- &EMR_NUM_INPUT and &EMR_CLASS_INPUT—refer to the input variables.
- &EMR_IMPORT_DATA—refers to the workflow data set.

Select the Code Editor ellipsis to create the R script as shown in Figure 8.6

**Figure 8.6: Code Editor**

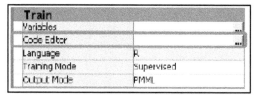

Program 8.7 shows an example of R script without variable handles, while Program 8.8 shows an example of R script with variable handles.

**Program 8.7: R Script Without Variable Handles**
```
&EMR_MODEL <- lm(rY ~ X1 + X2 + X3 +
C1 + C2 + C3, data =&EMR_IMPORT_DATA)
```

**Program 8.8: R Script With Variable Handles**
```
&EMR_MODEL <- lm(&EMR_NUM_TARGET ~
&EMR_NUM_INPUT + &EMR_CLASS_INPUT,
data=&EMR_IMPORT_DATA)
```

---

**Tip:** The &EMR_MODEL and &EMR_IMPORT_DATA variable handles must be used.

---

# Exercises

1. Choose the correct statements. Select all that apply.
   a. R can be called from Base SAS, SAS/IML, and SAS Enterprise Miner.
   b. -RLANG must be added to the SAS configuration file.
   c. PROC OPTIONS is used to test the SAS and R connection.
   d. You should leave SAS open when altering the configuration file.

2. The code below prints the first column of the data frame in the SAS Results Viewer.
```
call ExportDataSetToR("dog","rmatrix");
submit;
    rmatrix[,1]
endsubmit;
```
   a. True
   b. False

3. Variable handles must be used in SAS Enterprise Miner.
   a. True
   b. False

1. **Comparing Multiple Regression Estimates in SAS and R**
   a. Begin by invoking PROC IML and exporting the **fish** data set to R as a data frame with the name **Fish**.
   b. Fit a linear model with **Weight** as the dependent variable and **Height** and **Width** as the independent variables using the **lm()** function. Store the object and use the **summary()** function to print model estimates.
   c. Import the parameter estimates into an IML matrix. Recall that the parameter estimates are stored under the name **Coefficients** in the R object.
   d. Run the same analysis in SAS using PROC REG. Output the parameter estimates using the OUTEST= option in the PROC REG statement.
   e. Import the SAS coefficients into IML using the USE, READ, and CLOSE statements.
   f. Print the SAS coefficients and R coefficients side by side along with the difference between the estimates.

| SAS_COEFFICIENTS | R_COEFFICIENTS | DIFFERENCE |
|---|---|---|
| -433.6525 | -433.6525 | -5.12E-13 |
| 5.5068475 | 5.5068475 | -7.66E-13 |
| 177.44357 | 177.44357 | 1.648E-12 |

# Solutions

1. a, b, and c. You can call R from three separate environments: Base SAS using the DATA step, SAS/IML, and SAS Enterprise Miner using the Open Source Integration Node. In order for SAS and R to communicate you must add the –RLANG syntax to your SAS configuration file. Because SAS calls this file when you open a new session, you should close SAS when you make this change. To ensure SAS and R are connected you can use the OPTIONS procedure to test your connection.

2. b. Remember to use the / R option in the SUBMIT statement to send all code between the SUBMIT and ENDSUBMIT statements to R.

3. a. The object must be specified as &EMR_MODEL.

Programming Exercise

1. **Comparing Multiple Regression Estimates in SAS and R**

   a. Begin by invoking PROC IML and exporting the **fish** data set to R as a data frame with the name **Fish**.

   ```
   proc iml;
       call ExportDataSetToR("sp4r.fish","fish");
   ```

   b. Fit a linear model with **Weight** as the dependent variable and **Height** and **Width** as the independent variables using the **lm()** function. Store the object and use the **summary()** function to print model estimates.

   ```
   submit / r;
       fit <- lm(Weight ~ Height + Width, data=fish)
       summary(fit)
   endsubmit;
   ```

   ```
   Call:
   lm(formula = Weight ~ Height + Width, data = fish)

   Residuals:
       Min      1Q  Median      3Q     Max
   -249.90  -98.50  -46.03   57.34  890.57

   Coefficients:
                Estimate Std. Error t value Pr(>|t|)
   (Intercept) -433.653     37.020  -11.714   <2e-16 ***
   Height         5.507      5.086    1.083    0.281
   Width        177.444     12.884   13.773   <2e-16 ***
   ---
   Signif. codes:  0 '***' 0.001 '**' 0.01 '*' 0.05 '.' 0.1 ' ' 1

   Residual standard error: 166 on 155 degrees of freedom
     (1 observation deleted due to missingness)
   Multiple R-squared:  0.7891,    Adjusted R-squared:  0.7864
   F-statistic:   290 on 2 and 155 DF,  p-value: < 2.2e-16
   ```

   c. Import the parameter estimates into an IML matrix. Recall that the parameter estimates are stored under the name **Coefficients** in the R object.

   ```
   call ImportMatrixFromR(r_Coefficients,"fit$coefficients");
   ```

   d. Run the same analysis in SAS using PROC REG. Output the parameter estimates using the OUTEST= option in the PROC REG statement.

   ```
   submit;
       ods select none;
       proc reg data=sp4r.fish outest=sp4r.betas;
          model weight = height width;
       run; quit;
       ods select default;
   endsubmit;
   ```

e. Import the SAS coefficients into IML using the USE, READ, and CLOSE statements.

```
use sp4r.betas;
read all var {intercept height width} into sas_Coefficients;
close sp4r.betas;
```

f. Print the SAS coefficients and R coefficients side by side along with the difference between the estimates.

```
    coefficients = sas_coefficients` || r_coefficients ||
        (sas_coefficients` - r_coefficients);

    reset noname;
    coefficientNames = {SAS_Coefficients R_Coefficients
        Difference};
    print coefficients[colname=coefficientNames];
quit;
```

```
SAS_COEFFICIENTS R_COEFFICIENTS DIFFERENCE

       -433.6525      -433.6525  -5.12E-13
       5.5068475      5.5068475  -7.66E-13
       177.44357      177.44357  1.648E-12
```

# Ready to take your SAS® and JMP® skills up a notch?

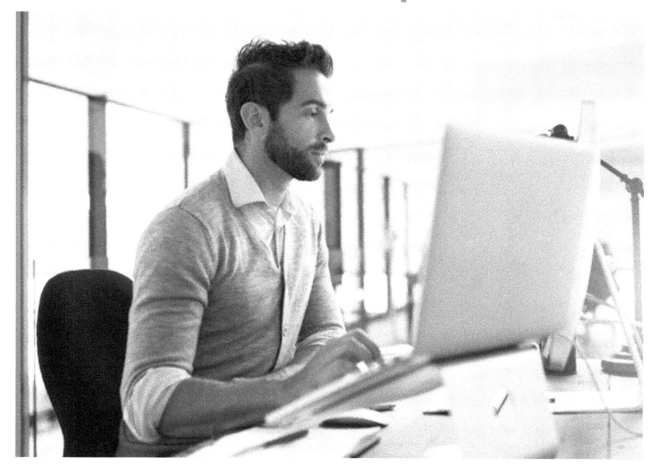

Be among the first to know about new books, special events, and exclusive discounts.
**support.sas.com/newbooks**

Share your expertise. Write a book with SAS.
**support.sas.com/publish**

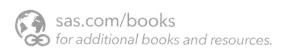

sas.com/books
*for additional books and resources.*

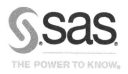

**THE POWER TO KNOW®**

www.ingramcontent.com/pod-product-compliance
Lightning Source LLC
Chambersburg PA
CBHW080635060326

40690CB00021B/4942